Annie Laurence SIKALI,
Selema AKEDJOL and Florence KISSOUGLE

Leisure activities amidst the COVID-19 health crisis

Preface by Maïgari BELLO BOUBA

L'Harmattan
Cameroun

5-7, rue de l'Ecole-Polytechnique, 75005 Paris

http://www.editions-harmattan.fr

ISBN : 978-2-14-026580-8
EAN : 9782140265808

Leisure activities amidst the COVID-19 health crisis

ACKNOWLEDGEMENTS

The publication of this training guide would not have been possible without the commitment of some personalities and the contribution of colleagues and collaborators in the Ministry of Tourism and Leisure.

Our sincere gratitude goes, first of all, to the Minister of State, Minister of Tourism and Leisure, BELLO BOUBA Maïgari, who, in implementing Government policy on tourism and leisure, instructed the organization of training seminars for youth leisure activity workers so as to adequately respond to the current national context of accelerated decentralization and the fight against the COVID-19 pandemic. We would also like to express our gratitude to Dr MANAOUDA Malachie, Minister of Public Health, who provided the workshops' organizing committee with a team of experts from his Ministry to educate participants on COVID-19 containment measures and ensure health coverage during the different sessions as well.

We would also like to thank Mr NDIORO A MAMOUM, Secretary General of the Ministry of Tourism and Leisure, for all the diligence and administrative coordination of the various workshops.

In like manner, we wish to fully appreciate the high collaborative spirit displayed by our colleagues throughout the implementation of these activities as well as the partners of the Ministry of Tourism and Leisure, most especially:

Finally, we express our profound gratitude to all those who have contributed in any way to the production of this book.

PREFACE

The year 2020 will be remembered in Cameroon and the world over as a year in which beliefs and practices were upset by the 2019 Corona Virus pandemic (COVID-19). As a matter of fact, tourism is one of the sectors of activity most affected by this health crisis, which has caused a general slowdown of services with the closure of recreational facilities, restrictions of people's movement, closure of borders and a drastic drop in tourism and leisure-related revenue.

Another major fact, not the least, however, is the speeding up of the decentralization process in the country. Indeed, Law No. 2019/024 of 24 December 2019 to lay down the general Decentralization Code sets out the organization of tourism and leisure activities as a devolved power, or one to be devolved more efficiently.

Decree No. 2012/291 of 21 June 2012 to organize the Ministry of Tourism and Leisure, extended the responsibility of our ministry. In line with this extended mission, in 2013 MINTOUL put in place strategies for the development and promotion of leisure activities through the organization of pilot holiday activities such as holiday camps, outdoor centres and youth camps.

Given the necessity to adapt to the current situation particularly marked by the fight against the COVID-19 pandemic, alongside the speeding up of the decentralization process, as well as the deployment of the extended powers of MINTOUL at institutional level, two major themes guided the training of holiday camp instructors for 2020 namely:

- How to organize leisure activities in a health crisis context like the COVID-19 pandemic;
- How to empower local and regional authorities to organize leisure activities.

To address these concerns, the trainers focused on the following objectives:

- Popularize the containment measures to be observed in order to prevent the spread of COVID-19 on account of the organization of tourist and leisure activities;
- Establish the code of conduct when faced with a suspected case of COVID-19 during a leisure activity;
- Increase the involvement of local and regional authorities in the development of tourism and leisure activities.

As can be observed, tourist and leisure activities cannot be organized on the basis of improvisation or amateurism. Moreover, it requires a strong ability to adjust to an ever-changing world.

As such, the ultimate purpose of the 2020 training session for leisure promoters was, first of all, to organize activities in strict compliance with hygiene and safety conditions, paying special attention to the full respect of containment measures and, secondly, to seize all the opportunities offered by decentralization, so as to provide Cameroonians with healthy and educative leisure activities. The knowledge acquired from this and previous training sessions would enable participants to carry out leisure activities with more confidence and serenity.

This publication, besides reiterating the technical and administrative conditions for organizing leisure activities, equally initiates reflection towards highlighting the challenges and opportunities that our political, social and cultural environment has to offer.

Maïgari BELLO BOUBA,

Minister of State,
Minister of Tourism and Leisure

FOREWORD

This guide was developed following a series of training sessions for leisure activity promoters held since 2018, at the Department of Leisure Development of the Ministry of Tourism and Leisure. The last training seminar for leisure activity promoters took place in the wake of the outbreak and spread of the Coronavirus pandemic. In addition, the pace of the decentralization process across the national territory was taken into account throughout the workshops.

The last participatory workshop was also in keeping with the measures implemented by the Ministry of Tourism and Leisure, in strict compliance with Government's approach for a global and effective response to the spread of the COVID-19 pandemic. Hinged decisively on the implementation of the decentralization process, this workshop was attended by representatives of local and regional authorities as well as civil society organizations, who followed with keen interest the issue of modalities of devolving powers to regional and local authorities for accelerated local development in the field of leisure.

The production of the publication in your hands, dear readers, was to a large extent, the outcome of the major recommendations from participants who followed the presentations of experts and participated in ensuing discussions. Documentary references alongside the legal and regulatory framework for leisure activities in Cameroon gave added value to the content.

Besides documentary sources, field experiences contributed greatly to the publication of this document, which is mostly a practical guide and intended primarily for leisure promoters.

Thus, one of the objectives of this guide is to provide partners of the tourism and leisure administration with a reference tool which is necessary for healthy and educative leisure activities, in accordance with the law and regulations. This is especially so as, in the effective implementation of Law No. 2019/024 of 24 December 2019 to lay down the general Code of Local and Regional Authorities, the Ministry of Tourism and Leisure is called upon to devolve certain powers to local authorities in the field of leisure. To this end, the supervisory authorities deemed it appropriate to support the publication of a technical and didactic document aimed at building the intervention capacities of public and private leisure activity promoters.

This handbook covers four aspects: first, it handles the regulations and techniques for organizing leisure activities in Cameroon; next, it highlights the measures for the prevention and fight against COVID-19; third, it focuses on the implementation of decentralization in the tourism and leisure sector, and rounds off with practical recommendations for the organization of healthy and educative leisure activities.

Annie Laurence SIKALI

Director of Leisure Development

INTRODUCTION

Since December 2019, the spread of the COVID-19 pandemic has held the attention of the entire world, causing widespread panic with its death toll and the uncertainty of finding a viable treatment or vaccine. Almost every sector has been affected worldwide, and in most cases this unexpected situation has brought about a chain of unpredictable and dramatic consequences.

One of the sectors most affected by this multidimensional crisis is that of tourism and leisure. In fact, observance of physical distancing measures, closure of recreational facilities, travel restrictions and the closure of borders make leisure activities almost impossible. Besides the financial losses incurred, isolation, restriction of freedom and psychological stress inflict immeasurable damage on individuals and communities. Multiple and prolonged confinement periods have disastrous consequences on the standard of living of individuals and communities owing to the drastic severance of social ties.

It should be noted that long before the health crisis, the leisure sector was already afflicted by other ills such as ignorance of regulations, inadequate supervisory staff as well as material and financial resources. Before the COVID-19 pandemic, the absence or insufficient practice of sports and leisure activities was already a factor of some malfunction in the society. Indeed, reliable studies suggest that some ills such as violence, drug addiction, juvenile delinquency and even some diseases are caused by the absence or insufficiency of healthy and educative leisure activities.

Disregard for regulations, inadequacy of human, material and financial resources, coupled with the COVID-19 crisis, are worsening factors in the crisis affecting the tourism and leisure sector. In other words, if the basic rules and techniques for organizing leisure activities are not mastered, practice will remain low and citizens' standards of living, precarious. In this context, if nothing is done, the COVID-19 crisis will just constitute another threat to the development of the leisure sector and citizens' standard of living.

Our concern is therefore how to sustain the promotion of leisure activities amidst a health crisis, notably the Coronavirus pandemic. What does the future hold for the leisure sector after the COVID-19 crisis? This book is thus divided into four chapters, titled as follows:

- The conceptual framework of leisure organization. This chapter includes definitions, laws and regulations, as well as the different techniques of leisure organization;
- The second chapter deals with practical examples for conducting some leisure activities;
- The third chapter focuses on general information on COVID-19, containment measures and protective equipment for caretakers;
- Finally, the fourth chapter deals with the future of leisure activities in the post-COVID-19 period.

CHAPTER I:

CONCEPTUAL FRAMEWORK OF LEISURE IN CAMEROON

The first chapter of this book focuses basically on the conceptual framework of leisure activities and revolves around four sections, namely:

- Regulatory framework of leisure activities;
- Definition of leisure;
- Types of leisure activities;
- Techniques for organizing leisure activities.

I. REGULATORY FRAMEWORK

Since independence, leisure activity control in Cameroon has been governed by regulatory texts. However, since 2011, the organization of leisure activities has been the responsibility of the Ministry of Tourism and Leisure. Prior to that, this responsibility had been entrusted to several other ministries, notably the Ministry of Youth and Sports or the Ministry of National Education.

As regards the regulatory framework, without being exhaustive, the following can be cited:

- Law No. 74/22 of 5 December 1974 on sports and socio-educational facilities;
- Law No. 2016/006 of 18 April 2016 to regulate tourism and leisure activities in Cameroon.

- Decree No. 2012/291 of 21 June 2012 to organize the Ministry of Tourism and Leisure;
- Order No. 2/CG/JS/EP of 15 February 1963 to regulate the organization and functioning of Holiday Camps in the Federal Republic of Cameroon.

The relevance of these texts, chosen on purpose, is to demonstrate that the leisure activities are a citizen's right and must be organized within a framework which targets the education, development and health of the citizen for their full participation in the development of the nation.

Law No. 2016/006 of 18 April 2016 to regulate tourism and leisure activities in Cameroon states in particular that:

- Article 5 : "The government, alongside the regional and local authorities, shall be responsible for implementing the national tourism and leisure policy."
- Article 6 : "Every natural person or legal entity has the right to carry out tourism and leisure activities over the territory, pursuant to the laws and regulations in force, and the standards of professionalism recognized by international norms and standards."

In accomplishing its missions, the Ministry of Tourism and Leisure has been organizing regular activities such as holiday camps, excursions and class outings since 2012. MINTOUL equally trains private sponsors of leisure activities and representatives of local and regional authorities. As a matter of fact, conducting these activities requires expertise that those in charge do not always have, particularly in the decentralized services. Moreover, from field observation, there is a general lack of qualified personnel among promoters and associations in the leisure sector.

The objective of the various training courses is therefore to equip stakeholders to meet the technical and operational requirements of leisure activities. More particularly, this involves making the organization of leisure activities more compliant with educational, hygiene and safety standards. The objective here is to give the population the widest possible access to activities, practice grounds and recreational services, and to contribute to well-being and improved standards of living.

The implementation of the texts in force and the achievements of the various training courses made it possible to arrive at some simplified but effective procedures that can be summed up in the steps here below.

Organizers of a leisure activity, whoever they may be (public or private bodies, associations, sports clubs), must comply with five major requirements:

- Declare the activity to MINTOUL;
- Respect supervision conditions during the activity;
- Define an educational project and a pedagogic project;
- Be covered by a civil liability insurance;
- Respect hygiene and safety rules.

On the basis of this protocol, many associations and companies have opened leisure centres and carousels, such as *Inter Progres* at the Conference Centre, Eco Park or "*La Forêt Enchantée* [The Enchanted Forest]" in the Bastos neighbourhood. In addition to training the staff of these private companies, the Ministry of Tourism and Leisure carries out inspection to monitor and control their activities.

In fact, Article 7 of the 2016 law states that: "Engaging in commercial and industrial tourism or leisure activities is subject, as the case may be, to first obtaining an authorization, an approval or a licence issued by the competent administration in charge of tourism and leisure…"

As regards implementing the above-mentioned measures, the Ministry of Tourism and Leisure is responsible for the inspection of leisure activities organized by the State or third parties. As provided for in Order No. 2/CG/JS/EP of 15 February 1963 to regulate the organization and operation of Holiday Camps in the Federal Republic of Cameroon, "Inspectors, thus nominated, may at any time enter the centres, in order to verify the number of people present, assess the comfort of the facilities, the educational value of the staff and the accounting documents."

In case of infringement, the supervision team has the power to apply the following sanctions:

- Warning ;
- Suspension of those in charge;
- Immediate closure of the camp;
- Withdrawal of subsidy, if applicable;
- Prohibition to reopen the camp the following year.

In case of emergency, the Ministry of Tourism and Leisure can order the immediate closure of a camp or leisure centre and take all the necessary measures for the dispersal of the children and their return to their families.

The Ministry of Tourism and Leisure in turn has already organized about twenty holiday camps, two each year. The last two editions took place in Baham and Bertoua, in strict compliance with the COVID-19 containment measures.

II. DEFINITION OF LEISURE

Leisure is generally understood to be « l'activité que l'on pratique durant le temps libre dont on peut disposer. Ce temps libre exclut le temps de travail et le temps de repos tels que l'emploi, les activités domestiques, l'éducation des enfants ou même le sommeil. » [an activity practiced during one's free time. This free time excludes work time and rest time activities such as one's job, domestic chores, children's education or even sleep] (Larousse Dictionary). Leisure is also referred to as "free time", that is time usually devoted to activities that are essentially non-productive from a macroeconomic point of view and often recreational.

According to Laurent TURCOT (2016), in his book on the history of sports and leisure, in ancient Greece, leisure activities and games were associated with royalty. Actually, entertainment was an activity reserved for free men, while slaves were reduced to roles of labourers or roles of arena beasts. Gladiators, who were generally slaves or convicts, were called upon to fight each other or fight ferocious beasts, to the delight of the upper class. Seneca regards leisure as the characteristic of the truly free man. The nobleman was more interested in free activity than in strenuous activity, in this case work, which was reserved for people of lower status.

The Industrial Revolution of the 18th and 19th centuries was characterized by the creation of factories where workers toiled for long hours for the mass production of goods and services. This situation led the International Labour Conference in Geneva in 1924 to sign a Convention on working hours, in order to guarantee workers, in addition to the necessary hours of sleep, sufficient time for leisure. In his book that analyses the relationship between work, leisure and social relations, Paul YONNET (1999) states that leisure activities contribute to the worker's balance and performance. In addition, leisure activities help to strengthen social relations and improve the social climate within the company.

Joffre DUMAZEDIER, a French sociologist (1915-2002), was the first to take real interest in leisure activities for scientific research and gave it a more in-depth definition. For him, leisure activities are "a set of occupations to which the individual can devote himself/herself voluntarily either to relax, to be entertained, or to develop through information or disinterested training, his/her voluntary social participation or his/her free creative capacity after breaking free from his/her professional, family and social obligations." He develops the idea according to which leisure activities must have three purposes: to relax, to be entertained and to develop (RED).

- Relaxation relieves fatigue and overwork;
- Entertainment is a way of enjoying oneself and fighting against boredom and the negative effects of the division of labour;
- Development of personality corresponds to one's time for social, cultural and sporting participation, as well as practical activities.

The trend towards leisure civilization as described by DUMAZEDIER has led to the creation of leisure industries and even a leisure economy. The term "leisure industry" refers to goods and services, which satisfy the needs of individuals and groups in terms of tourist activities or destinations.

The role of leisure activities as an element of public health, development and social cohesion is now more recognised than ever. The benefits of leisure and physical activities are well established in terms of physical health and psychological well-being. They are notably reflected in the academic motivation of young people, the productivity of workers, the independence of the elderly and the development of communities.

In the context of Cameroon and according to the Law of 18 April 2016 to regulate tourism and leisure activities in Cameroon, a leisure activity refers to any "physical, recreational, sporting, cultural, intellectual or scientific activity organized for the sole purpose of relaxation, entertainment or development of one's abilities."

III. TYPES OF LEISURE ACTIVITIES

There are countless leisure activities related to sport, culture, relaxation, games, adventure, discovery, creativity, art work, etc.

1. Sporting activities

Sport is no longer just a matter of the elite or for winning prizes. The practice of sport is becoming more democratic and even popular, meaning that it is practised by people from all walks of life who are not much interested in performance. Practising a sport regularly like walking or jogging alone or in a group, going to the gym, cycling, or participating in "two zero" has become quite popular in our neighbourhoods and villages. There are a thousand and one ways to combine sport and leisure, whether it is practiced in a leisure centre with animation or on one.

Sporting activities have unimaginable benefits such as facilitating daily life, protecting against chronic diseases, improving sleep quality, fighting stress, etc. This is the goal of the Cameroon Federation of Sport for All, which promotes the democratic practice of leisure activities.

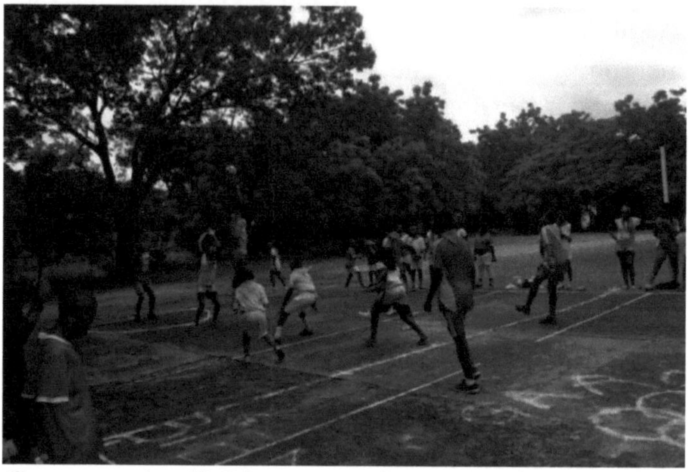

Game scene in a Holiday camp in Garoua, North region (D.R.).

2. Cultural activities

Going to the cinema or theatre, learning to play a musical instrument or taking dancing classes are activities that particularly attract young people during their free time. Cultural activities include a wide range of activities like drawing, carving, pottery, jewellery making, decoration, etc. Meanwhile, music helps to reduce anxiety, improve self-esteem and give a considerable sense of control over one's life. Some schools and even private institutions offer arts and culture training to young people and adults to improve their memory.

Participating in the writing of a newspaper or hosting a radio programme, surfing the net to discover a wide range of information are some of the activities young people do in their free time. By themselves or under guidance from school authorities, they organize karaoke, video game competitions or street dance caravans. In Senegal for example, street painting is a fast-growing phenomenon. Unfortunately, there is a drop in the number of people who still read and go to the cinema in Cameroon and in Africa in general.

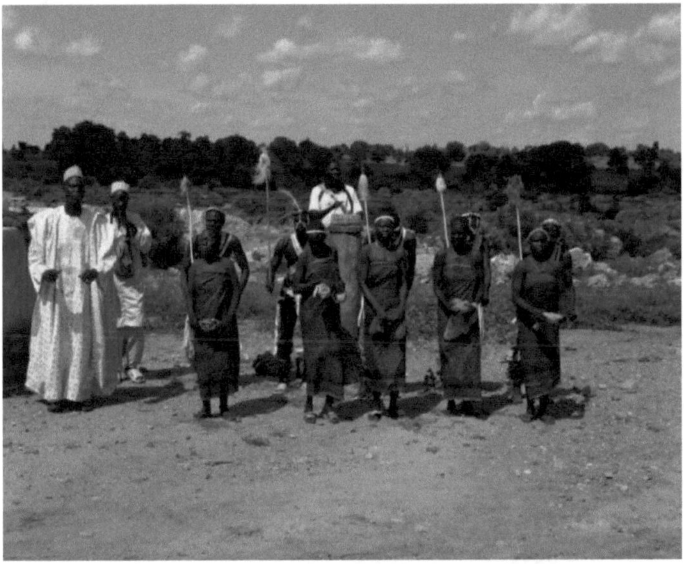

Lamà dance, Guider, North region (D.R.).

3. Creative leisure activities

Besides the common cultural activities, there are other thought creative activities such as writing books, comics, plays, or painting landscapes. With the development of IT, we have witnessed the creation of designs in different fields like fashion, advertising and even architecture. Instilling creativity into one's life contributes to mental balance and health. Apart from putting one in the best of moods, it helps to improve well-being.

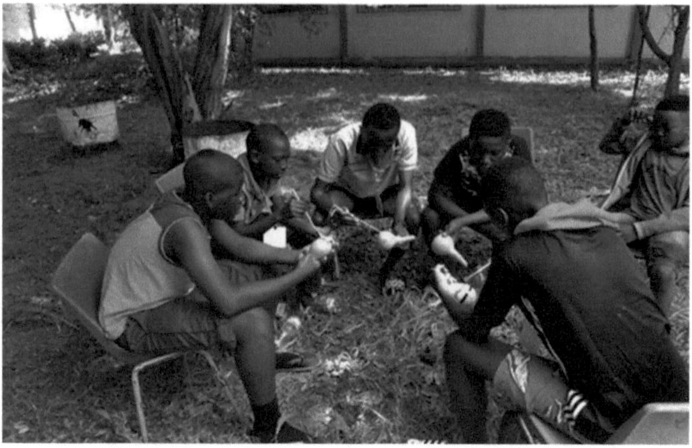

Training on how to paint calabashes (D.R.).

4. Outdoor activities

Walking is known to be beneficial after hard work or a prolonged quarantine period. Excursions in the woods, on mountains or at the beach do not only build stamina and self-control, but also give pleasure and the opportunity to discover new landscapes. Visiting botanic or animal parks improves one's knowledge of different species and helps discover the secrets of nature.

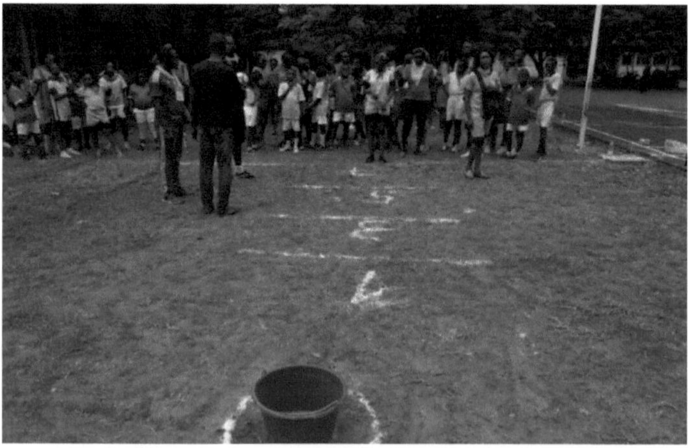

Ready for a game of skill played with a bucket (D.R.).

5. Discovery leisure activities

Discovery leisure activities include travel, excursions, explorations, expeditions, etc. It is about going in search of new landscapes and cultures, with the aim not only of enjoying oneself, as well as opening up to other realities. Such adventures can take place in the natural environment, in the city, in developed areas and even, increasingly, virtually. These leisure activities also include discoveries in the scientific field, as long as they are not work-related.

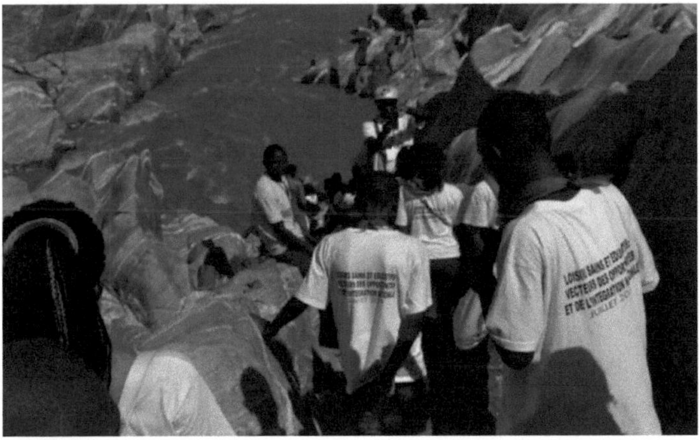

Visiting the "Kola Gorges" tourist site near Guider, North region (D.R.).

6. Board games

There are several other forms of recreational activities that have been grouped under “board games”. These are games that used to be played in parlours, but have now become popular. These include draughts, scrabble, ludo and monopoly. Nowadays, these games include billiards, pinball, table football, etc. They also include some traditional games such as Songo, Wari-wari or Awale. It should be noted that playing these games compulsively can lead to unhealthy addictions.

7. Specific leisure activities

Some other forms of leisure activities can be called specific because they are similar to normal activities. For example, cooking, gardening or bricolage can, in some ways, be considered as work. There is a class of people who greatly enjoy doing these activities without feeling any discomfort or reluctance. Others also engage in activities like first aid or humanitarian work, without expecting any compensation.

It is worth mentioning that the classification of leisure activities can only be indicative, as they are not only interrelated, but also evolve with time and the environment. One really has to travel around the world to discover the diversity of leisure activities. Let us now focus on the specific case of Cameroon.

IV. TECHNIQUES FOR ORGANIZING LEISURE ACTIVITIES

Techniques for organizing leisure activities are closely related to the types of activities and the educational projects of the promoters. These educational projects, as well as the consequent activities, depend themselves, on a number of factors which include the environment, culture, infrastructure, educational objectives, age of participants, etc. The educational project is therefore specific to the characteristics of each type of activity. It expresses the collective commitment of a pedagogic team within a given time and environment and serves as reference throughout the action concerned. It is a “contract of trust” established between the manager of the accommodation centre, the pedagogic team, external stakeholders and the children’s parents. It gives meaning to the proposed activities and helps to build a pedagogic approach based on objectives and including an evaluation method.

In any case, the organization of leisure activities responds to a questionnaire structured around the following concerns:

- Which activity should be chosen and for which target group?
- What are the objectives ?
- What is the best time to organize the activity?
- What is the best place to organize the activity?
- What means should be mobilized to organize the activity?

Promoters will have to choose the most appropriate and feasible activity, based on the answers obtained. In their elaborate form, leisure activities can be organized in different forms, such as:

- Clubs ;
- Walks, excursions and picnics;
- Holiday championships;
- Caravans and festivals ;
- Youth camps ;
- Youth villages and holiday villages;
- Holiday camps.

1. Clubs

Clubs are forms of association or circles built around intellectual, sporting, cultural or recreational activities. They are specific activities practised in conjunction with broader activities. Generally, they are based on a collective and individual commitment to a cause or a passion (environmental protection, promotion of a language, intergenerational solidarity, humanitarian work, etc.). In schools, such examples as “press clubs”, “health clubs” or “nature clubs” are common.

2. Walks, excursions and picnics

Walks, excursions and picnics are outings organized around a theme. The objectives and means must be specified before departure. It can be about discovering nature or visiting buildings like monuments or museums. The necessary attire, equipment and provisions should be carefully prepared. Usually, a guide is needed to explain the history, culture and functioning of the places visited.

3. Holiday championships

Holiday championships refer to the gathering of young people for sporting activities for entertainment purposes. Very often, they are combined with cultural and engagement activities targeting social or national interests. The purpose here is not really performance and competition, but having fun and bringing young people together. However, a holiday championship that is only based on games quickly becomes boring. There must therefore always be an educational objective for behavioural change. The holiday championship can also be a powerful means of mobilizing young people to raise their awareness on specific concerns, for example the fight against the ills that undermine the youth or the promotion of civic values.

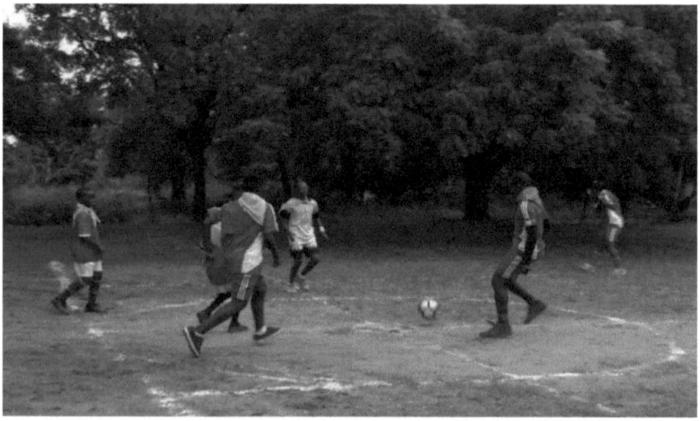

Football match during a holiday championship (D.R.).

4. Caravans and festivals

Caravans and festivals are activities that take place intermittently in different places. Examples include group travel based on a specific subject or cause, such as culture or humanitarian work.

Caravans are travelling activities that involve participants going from place to place either to perform or discover the tourist and cultural realities of a given area. Participants in caravans generally travel in converted vehicles called "caravans", which serve as light housing or mobile leisure homes.

Festivals, on the other hand, are cultural and/or artistic events organized at well specific places and periods. They can either be traditional or modern. Among Cameroon's most renown traditional festivals, can be cited the NGUON of the Bamouns and the NGONDO of the Doualas. As far as modern music is concerned, the "*Festi Bikutsi*" and « *Jazz sous les manguiers* » [Jazz under the mango trees] are noteworthy. Objectives of festivals include the discovery of new forms of expression and disclosure of a message from the custodians of tradition.

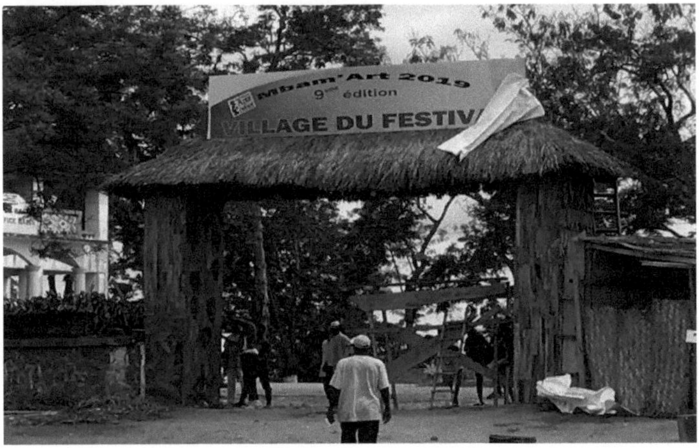

Entrance of the Mbam'Art Festival site in Bafia, Centre region (D.R.).

5. Youth camps

Youth camps are a kind of mobilizations for young people aged 16 and above, around a physical exercise, notably the construction or restoration of a facility. It may also be a forum for learning or testing skills. Youth camps seek to facilitate interaction between young people from different backgrounds, working together to restore a locality or to help people. The youth volunteer camp can concern such diverse areas as architectural heritage, the environment, rehabilitation of houses or small socio-educational or sports facilities. Although the programme of the come together may be focused on the camp's project, it also encourages inter-cultural, even international encounter involving persons from different backgrounds. The International Organization of *la Francophonie* encourages the movement of young people in the French-speaking world through youth camps.

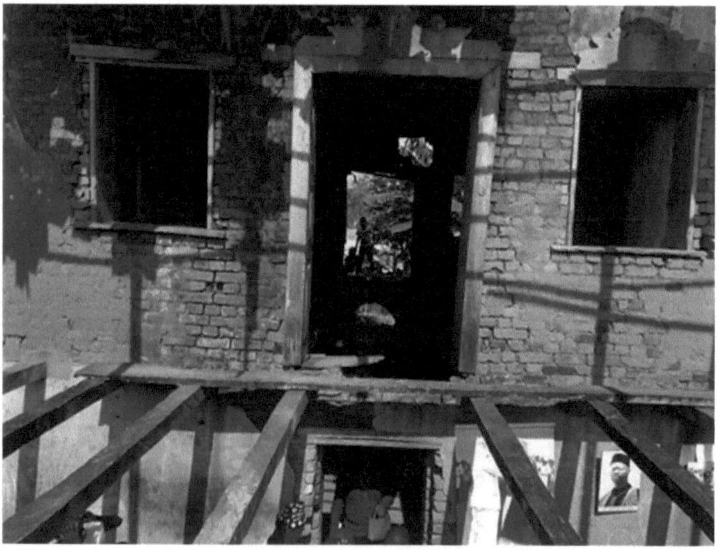

Excursion and visit to a historic building in Bafia, Centre region (D.R.).

6. Holiday villages

Holiday villages are accommodation centres for groups from different backgrounds for cultural discovery, entertainment, relaxation and development of human relations. They are different from traditional hotels in that the promoters provide the setting, while the holiday-makers themselves organize their lives and stay there.

They are places where people of all ages and social status meet, work and live together during their stay. Together, they build a world that is open to change and that respects individual values.

However, the internal rules and regulations which are made known to all must be observed by each resident of the holiday village, particularly as regards hygiene and safety.

7. Holiday camps

The holiday camp has been the main activity to be successfully organized by the Ministry of Tourism and Leisure for almost a decade now. This is why we would like to focus on its organizational technique, which is one of the most complex.

Holiday camps or "Holiday and Leisure Centres with Lodging" are Collective Accommodation for Minors organized around an educational project, and take place during school holidays or leisure time. They must comply with the regulations and standards in force and are directed and run by qualified staff, under the supervision of State services.

They generally last between 5 and 21 days and are held in buildings or tents. Hygiene and safety measures must be strict, likewise the requirement of an educational project drawn up by qualified persons. A holiday camp is also characterized by regulatory requirements pertaining to the physical setting, educational project and health measures.

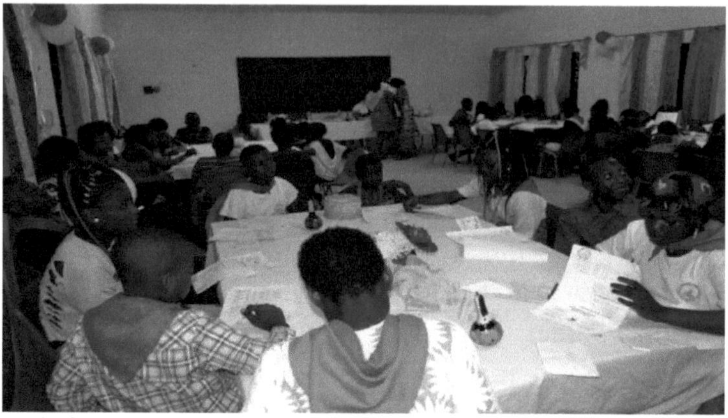

End of camp assessment by the participants in Bertoua, East region (D.R.).

7.1. Physical setting

The premises that host minors during a holiday camp are subject to strict regulation. Their objective should be to ensure comfort and safety for all. It is the operator's responsibility to register the premises used, and to maintain it in optimal hygiene and safety conditions. The area hosting a holiday camp must be easily accessible to the various rescue services (hospital, police, gendarmerie, fire-fighters, etc.) in case of danger, accident or illness. The premises must be accessible to movement impaired persons, and under normal conditions of use. In accordance with the regulations in force, camp organizers are obliged to host the children in premises that meet strict hygiene and safety conditions.

Safety requirements are determined by the equipment, accommodation capacity and ranking of the facility in question. For example, here are the major measures to be respected for a 50-person capacity holiday centre:

- The facility must have at least two exits;
- The site must have an adequate security lighting system;
- The spaces must be partitioned according to activities to be carried out (dormitory, refectory, infirmary, playgrounds, etc.);
- A notice relating to the care of persons with disabilities.

The entire premises (activity halls, dining hall, kitchens, toilets, bathrooms, dormitories, etc.) must be adequately ventilated to ensure sufficient air exchange, in accordance with the regulations. Ventilation eliminates pollutants from human presence, as well as odours and moisture from condensation. Natural lighting must be prioritized in the main rooms so that activities are carried out without using artificial lighting.

The dormitory must have attached to it:

- 1 toilet for 10 or less persons;
- A bathroom or individual cabins, that is 1 shower head for 10 or less persons;
- 1 sink for 5 persons.

As far as possible, the facilities should be connected to water, electricity and telephone networks. In the absence of a public connection, waste water must be treated in a non-public treatment system adapted to the capacity of the facility.

The space meant to host holiday camps must have ample spaces for cultural, manual and sports activities. If necessary, the animation team should make sure that these areas are put in order before each session.

Facilities meant to host leisure activities must strictly comply with hygiene and safety rules. Safety requirements shall be determined by the layout, accommodation capacity and the type of activities to be carried out. Technical facilities (water, electricity, gas, etc.) must be checked to ensure that they function properly before the site opens. In any case, whatever the structure of the facility and its accommodation capacity, prior inspection should validate the choice of facility before the start of activities.

7.2. Gender diversity and social inclusion

Camps with accommodation must be organized in such a way that girls and boys above the age of six may sleep in separate areas. Each minor must have their sleeping bag.

The law on the protection of persons with disabilities reiterates the principle of free accessibility for all. Hosting children collectively requires that everyone, regardless of their disability or health condition, should participate in activities to the best of their abilities. The aim is to ease the integration of each child with other children of the same age, while adjusting, at a young age, their perception of disability. This approach requires that the organizers, director and youth activity workers, should have been informed before the camp on the specific disabilities of the child(ren). The supervisory team must also be well informed on the precautions to take to guarantee the well-being of the children and their participation in activities.

7.3. Supervision conditions

Taking care of many children at the same time requires some level of organization or even expertise. It should be noted that no matter the dexterity and experience of a youth activity worker, they cannot efficiently follow up children above a certain number. It is therefore necessary to set the number of children per supervisor. The following essential criteria must be strictly respected when organizing a holiday camp:

- The number of participants: at least 7 children;
- Age of participants: between 3 and 16 years (the age difference between children of the same group should be 4 years maximum);
- Duration of the camp: between 5 and 21 days;
- A highly qualified staff should be in charge of the management: Certificate for youth activity worker (BAFA) or an equivalent;
- Supervision must be carried out by duly trained persons (Youth Activity Workers and Intern Youth Activity Workers);
- The number must be respected: 1 youth activity worker for 8 children below 6 years or 1 youth activity worker for 12 children of 6 years and above.

7.4. Educational project

The promoter of a holiday camp must submit their educational project at the time with the declaration. This document must include the psychological and physiological needs of the children to be hosted, that should be met through the community life and practice of the various activities organized. The educational project sets the objectives of the educational activity, specifying the measures for its implementation. It must be communicated to the children's parents before departure so that they know beforehand what skills will be required, as well as the values that will be instilled in their children.

This document shall describe, in particular, the nature of activities offered, the different moments and time allocated to each activity and to rest respectively. In any case, an activity timetable must be provided in advance. It may be changed or modified depending on the constraints of the field, without any fundamental change in its original objective.

The educational objective is the main focus of every holiday camp. This objective states the educational intentions of the organizer, and is implemented pedagogically by the team of youth activity workers. It takes into account the psychological and physiological needs of the children, as well as environmental conditions, accordingly adjusting the organization of the holiday camp. The inherent educational objective of every holiday camp includes teamwork and the exemplary nature of all supervisors. The pedagogic project gives meaning to the organized activities and community life. It serves as reference and ensures that the children or young people can blossom in an environment where the physical and moral integrity of all is guaranteed.

The educational objectives on the other hand, highlight the cross-cutting objectives of all the actions carried out by the organizer. For example:

- Enable children from less privileged backgrounds to go on holiday;
- Foster meetings between young people from different areas and backgrounds;
- Develop the integration of children with mild disabilities during camps with able-bodied young people;
- Help boys and girls to mingle in the quarters;
- Raise the awareness of minors on environmental issues and promote sustainable development;
- Promote inter cultural exchange through games.

These educational objectives must correspond to the needs expressed by families and young people, in conjunction with local elected representatives and community leaders in the area in question. These objectives should be sustainable, if possible, taking into account the social context and local dynamics.

Ultimately, an educational objective should be Specific, Measurable, Attainable, Realistic and Time-bound (SMART). The programme of planned activities must be implemented in accordance with pedagogic objectives and possibilities offered. These activities should be varied, suited to the age and intellectual, physical and creative abilities of the children, and must be properly supervised.

As far as possible, we must listen to young people if we intend to build them into a “source of initiative” and win their collaboration. It is also recommended having several activities, with the possibility to switch from one to another. It is wise to plan alternative activities in case of bad weather, an obstruction or failure.

Where physical or sporting activities requiring specialized supervision are planned, the pedagogic project must specify the supervision that will be provided on this occasion. The day-to-day planning of activities during the stay will determine the timetable of the youth activity workers. It is important to plan activities daily, because it is a good indicator of the camp’s level of preparation. It is one of the main documents to present during an inspection. This planning should include the following aspects :

- Organization of toileting (use of showers, supervision procedures, respect for the children’s privacy, etc.);
- Organization of meals (proposed menu, prohibitions for religious or medical reasons, etc.);
- Time management (activity and rest time, respect of the rhythms according to the age and needs of each

child, wake-up time bedtime, evening entertainment, etc.);

- Modalities for children's participation (freedom of expression, sharing of experiences and resolutions, etc.);
- Respect and/or organization of religious activities;
- Health monitoring of minors (pharmacy, medicines management and follow up of children under treatment, etc.);
- Family information (post office box, email and telephone access, etc.);
- Camp rules, or non-negotiable rules that apply to the whole group;
- Sanctions provided for in case of breach;
- The schedule of a typical day.

Finally, the pedagogic project must include camp assessment methods. The assessment process seeks to understand the success factors as well as reasons for any difficulties encountered during the camp, and hence, to analyse the relevance of the action taken. Assessment is a daily process and is the main purpose of the supervision team meetings. At the end of the camp, it is necessary to draft a global assessment record of the project, with all the players: team of youth activity workers, children, parents, organizers, partners, public authorities, etc.

7.5. The medical certificate, pharmacy and infirmary

Before each child leaves for the holiday camp, their parents must provide a medical certificate signed by a State doctor. Information about the child's health may also be required: vaccination status, allergies or medical treatment. The staff and each person working in the camp must also provide proof of their health condition (medical certificate, COVID-19 test, etc.).

The medical certificate is a key document in preparations for a camp with young people. Apart from being compulsory, it enables families communicate important information about the child's health condition to the group leader or health assistant. It is therefore crucial that the medical certificate be filled with objectivity and transparency by a sworn doctor. In the event of an accident or illness, it helps the group leader or the health assistant to have and immediately provide health professionals with the necessary information for an immediate and effective treatment of the child.

The presence of a health assistant is compulsory in all camps or trips involving minors. This person must be at least a qualified nurse. They are responsible for the health supervision and monitoring of everyone in the group, including supervisors. Their role is mainly to:

- Organize the infirmary and manage daily "small" routine care;
- Give first aid and organize rescue in the event of an accident;
- Collect, check and keep medical certificates;
- Ensure the physical and psychological well-being of the children and listen to them;
- Make children and supervisors aware of possible risks;
- Liaise with parents in the event of an accident or illness affecting a child.

It is strictly forbidden for a supervisor to give medication to a minor without due prescription by a doctor. Medication is never to be administered haphazardly. It must suit a specific case; a badly followed dosage or an unknown allergy can have dramatic consequences.

To deal with minor injuries, each holiday camp must have a small pharmacy set up with respect to the number of people in the group, the surrounding environment and the physical or sporting activities envisaged.

It is imperative for each camp with accommodation to have an infirmary, separate from the dormitory, where the sick can be taken in or a participant isolated to avoid cases of contamination.

7.6. Civil liability insurance

Proof of insurance coverage is an essential part of the holiday camp organization file. Holiday camp organizers, like the operator of the facility where the camp is held, are obliged to take out an insurance policy covering the financial consequences of their civil liability, as well as that of their employees and participants in the activities they offer. Organizers shall also inform the parents of the minors involved, of their intention to buy an insurance policy.

CHAPTER II:

PEDAGOGIC GUIDE FOR CONDUCTING LEISURE ACTIVITIES

The effective work of leisure activity promoters generally consists in preparing, organizing and evaluating scheduled socio-cultural, recreational or sporting activities. Understood as such, one might be tempted to believe it is a very simple task for anyone. But on closer observation, it is quite evident that the slightest negligence or ignorance of the rules can lead to failure and even dramatic situations. Practical organization of leisure activities requires all-round and thorough preparation. Be it at the level of venue choice, selection of the participants or adoption of the activity itself, everything must be prepared ahead of time to avoid any unpleasant surprises. Hence, it becomes needful to recall some practical recommendations for anyone seeking to engage in the organization of leisure activities. We will not be going back to the administrative formalities already addressed in the first chapter.

To illustrate our point, we will use three case studies:

- Organizing a sport walk;
- Managing a cultural festival ;
- Organizing a holiday camp.

I. ORGANIZING A SPORT WALK

Practised on a regular basis in small groups or during major events, sport walk has become a very highly valued activity for Cameroonians, especially among adults. Hiking or walking to keep fit or lose weight has become a popular activity throughout our towns and country sides. It is worth recalling that there are several types of walking techniques: simple walking, hiking, fast walking, Afghan walking, etc. Depending on the objectives, the promoter must define the target audience, the location, the equipment required, the route and the distance to be covered for the ideal organization of a walk. Regardless of the technique chosen and the objectives sought, a few compulsory rules must be observed to ensure that the walk is carried out following the required safety conditions.

Rule 1: Identify and secure the site or route

Walking can take place in the streets of a town, in the forest, in the mountains or on the beach. For each of these sites, appropriate measures must be taken.

If the walk is taking place inside town, for example, there should be:

- A signal at the head of the walk;
- A signal at the tail of the walk;
- A safety strip to separate walkers from the roadway where cars and other vehicles move.

If the walk is done in the countryside (forest, mountain, beach), it is recommended to:

- Mark out the route to make it easier to find the track to be followed;
- Have guides within the group to direct walkers;

- Provide mopping or water refreshment points or provide each walker with an individual kit;
- Have a rescue team available for those who might need help.

Rule 2: Define the participants

Who can take part in a sport walk? Walking is much more suitable for young people and adults than for children and teenagers, depending on their abilities and hobbies. It is also important to differentiate between experienced athletes and seasonal walkers. The former may become bored and the latter discouraged. It is therefore advisable to observe the following measures:

- Pick walkers from among people with similar levels of experience to facilitate group cohesion and effort control;
- Require basic medical tests (blood pressure, weight and temperature, COVID-19 test, etc.) to ensure that everyone is physically fit to take part in the activity.

Rule 3: Get the right equipment

What equipment is needed for the walk? Depending on the time and place of the activity, walkers should put on appropriate footwear and attire. Sports shoes should be chosen for their flexibility to avoid possible injuries. Clothing should be loose fitting to facilitate movement and perspiration without exposing the walker to dehydration.

The equipment (attire and footwear) should contribute to the safety and comfort of participants. As such, the following guidelines should be observed:

- Acquire shoes that suit the type of walking (rangers for hiking and trekking or trainers for walking);

- Choose the right shoe size (neither too big nor too small) to avoid blocking blood circulation and blisters;
- Wear loose, flexible clothes and tracksuits to facilitate movement;
- Equip walkers with a personal kit or provide refreshment points with water and other foods;
- Acquire emergency equipment to help people in distress (medical kit, water, compass, sleeping bag, ambulance, etc.).

Rule 4: Put in place a supervision team

A supervision team is necessary to ensure that the walk takes place in optimal safety conditions. A professional or trained supervisor knows the basic rules for practising a sporting activity and ensures that they are observed:

- Warm up before starting the walk to avoid contractures, tears and strains;
- Monitor speed in order to start smoothly and gain momentum;
- Decide on pace with respect to abilities and objectives (6 km/h is the average required);
- Calculate the duration of the effort (at least 30 to 45 minutes are necessary to produce effects);
- Stretch after the effort to reduce toxins (lactic acid) in the muscles;
- Massage legs to regulate circulation;
- Hydrate regularly;
- If possible, eat fruits and vegetables after the activity.

II. MANAGING A CULTURAL FESTIVAL

Organizing a cultural event like a festival, fair or concert for entertainment purposes requires thorough preparation and expertise. To achieve this, a questionnaire is recommended as a guideline. Which festival? For who? Why a festival? When to organize a festival? With what means should a festival be organized? The answers to these various questions have led us to discover ten (10) steps to organize a festival and similar cultural events.

Step 1: Define the theme of the festival

By definition, a festival is an artistic or cultural event organized periodically in a particular place or on a rotatory basis within a given area. There are therefore several types of festivals depending on the field, content and objectives pursued:

- Artistic festival: It is based on arts such as music, dance or theatre, with the aim of enhancing the culture of an area or promoting new styles;
- Heritage and poly-cultural festival: The aim is to highlight different facets of a culture in areas as varied as customs and traditions, gastronomy, dances, etc.;
- Economic festival: This has to do with exhibiting and selling the products of an area field of activity: agriculture, fishing, breeding, etc.

Step 2: Identify the setting for the activity

A festival can take place in the open air or in a closed environment; the most important thing for the organizer is to choose a setting that meets the best conditions as regards accessibility, hygiene and safety.

Step 3: Select players

Players should be picked from among the people best qualified to contribute to the theme of the festival, though this also depends on the means available. Needless asking for professional artists with small budgets when you could do with casual, amateurs or volunteer artists.

Step 4: Get the right equipment

For school socials in a school, one can use light equipment to cover a small area. But for large-scale events, comfort and listening conditions must be suitable.

Step 5: Draw up a calendar

When organizing a festival, one must take into account a number of contingencies like weather conditions, availability of space, stakeholders and even the target population. It is therefore necessary to identify the different tasks that contribute to the success of the event and put them in a timetable.

Step 6: Draft and determine the budget

The scope of the event must be in line with the resources available. You should not think too big or too small; it is simply a matter of being realistic. Many applications for subsidies are not successful because the budget requested is unrealistic. In addition, many initiatives fail because of a low budget in the course of the activity. In sum, it is important to know, beforehand, the cost of the project and its funding sources as well as their guarantee.

Step 7: Fulfil legal obligations

Depending on the size of the event, the promoter of a festival must obtain either an authorization or a declaration from competent authorities. Very often, authorities are only contacted when disputes or incidents occur. It then becomes difficult to determine who is responsible under such conditions. In such cases, that responsibility falls on the promoter of the event.

Step 8: Contact health and safety authorities

In addition to the administrative procedures described above, any public or private promoter of a festival must request security and health coverage during the event. Indeed, during mass events, no one is safe from a malaise, stampede or any other inconvenience. The assistance of the medical staff or the forces of law and order is therefore essential.

Step 9: Take out an insurance policy

As long as everything goes smoothly, everyone is safe. The importance of an insurance policy can be seen in case an incident occurs. Taking out an insurance policy is a compulsory measure for organizing a festival and any other mass event.

Step 10: Publicize the event

Informing the public is one of the keys to the success of a festival and any cultural event. It is in the interest of promoters to use both traditional and electronic media to advertise their events. The traditional means includes posters, banners, flyers, leaflets, as well as the radio, TV and press releases. Electronic media include social media (WhatsApp, Twitter, Facebook, etc.) or websites created for the activity.

Step 11: Remunerate the players

As mentioned at the time of budgeting, many activities end up in litigation due to non-compliance with the terms of reference, particularly with regard to the remuneration of players. For some, it is breach of trust, for others huge appetites; such is the daily reality of relations between artists and show sponsors. To protect the rights of both parties, it is advisable to sign a contract or a memorandum of understanding beforehand and honour it.

III. ORGANIZING A HOLIDAY CAMP

As mentioned in the first chapter, holiday camps are the flagship activity of the Department of Leisure Development of the Ministry of Tourism and Leisure. It is equally the activity for which subsidies are most applied by private leisure promoters. We therefore thought it would be useful to focus on rules to respect when organizing a holiday camp.

Step 1: State the theme of the holiday camp

The educational purpose should be clear from the statement of the theme of the camp and should be communicated to the parents so that they can easily grasp the values or skills that the organizer intends to instill in their children. The theme can be inspired by several factors (physical environment, culture, civic values, etc.).

Step 2: Meet legal obligations

For non-State organizations (association, private person), an approval or authorization from the Minister in charge of Tourism and Leisure is obligatory.

Step 3: Carry out an ex-ante inspection

The issue of the health and safety requirements in and around the premises where the holiday camps are to be held cannot be overemphasized. An inspection team from the Ministry of Tourism and Leisure or any other relevant authority should issue a clearance for a holiday camp site.

Step 4: Define participation conditions

Every organizer of a holiday camp must produce a document specifying participation conditions of young people. This includes criteria such as age, gender, origin, financial conditions, equipment required, etc.

Step 5: Form the supervision team

Forming here has a double meaning: the first involves providing supervisors with the knowledge essential for the organization of the holiday camp. The second involves putting together a dynamic and united team that will not only develop the educational and pedagogic project, but also set and enforce the rules of living in the camp.

Step 6: Draft the educational and pedagogic project

The educational and pedagogic project is a derivative of the camp theme. It should include, in detail, the planning of activities and rules of living in the camp. It is not just a simple timetable. It is a document that incorporates the objectives, timing, sequences, as well as the methods and activities to attain the objectives.

Step 7: Set up a technical team

Apart from the supervisors and children, many other people intervene in the camp (medical staff, cleaners, cooks, etc.) These people must be chosen according to the size of the camp, but also with regard to their skills and moral integrity.

Step 8: Select participants

For several reasons, it may happen that not all the children who apply for a camp are selected (limited number of places, non-compliance with admission conditions, etc.). In any case, the final list of children selected must be known for other administrative formalities (insurance, medical check-ups, inspections, travel, etc.).

Step 9: Take out an insurance policy

Every organizer of a holiday camp (State or private sponsor) must take out an insurance policy to cover all participants. This insurance covers the children and supervisors, as well as support staff.

Step 10: Seek security coverage

Violence and terrorism are realities which we will have to live with for a while. Besides, anyone can fall victim to an accident, robbery or kidnapping. With such apprehensions, it is essential to inform the authorities beforehand of the organization of a holiday camp in their area of jurisdiction.

Step 11: Ensure the transportation of participants to and from the camp

Transportation of children to and from the camp or during outings must be carried out in optimal safety conditions.

CHAPTER III:

LEISURE ACTIVITIES AND HEALTH CRISIS
EXPERIENCE WITH THE COVID-19 PANDEMIC
HYGIENE AND CONTAINMENT MEASURES AGAINST COVID-19

I. GENERAL INFORMATION ON COVID-19

1. Definition

COVID-19 or the Coronavirus disease 2019 is an infectious and contagious disease caused by a virus called coronavirus. It was first identified in humans in Wuhan, central China in December 2019. The symptoms of the disease range from the common cold to more severe illnesses.

2. Epidemiological significance

In December 2019, COVID-19 was reported in Wuhan, central China. It spread very rapidly throughout the world and, on 30 January 2020, was declared by the WHO as a Public Health Emergency of International Concern (PHEIC). On 11 March 2020, it became a pandemic with a 2.6% mortality rate.

3. Mode of transmission

COVID-19 is transmitted directly or indirectly through respiratory droplets.

3.1. Direct transmission

Respiratory droplets from a carrier of the virus when they cough or sneeze directly infect a healthy person.

3.2. Indirect transmission

The transfer of the infectious agent is done from a reservoir to a host. Transmission occurs through contact with soiled objects or surfaces, and then contact with the eyes, nose or mouth.

Airborne transmission occurs when infectious agents are carried by dust or airborne droplet nuclei. Carriers can indirectly transmit the infectious agent. The vector can transmit the infectious agent or promote its growth or change.

3.3. Incubation

Incubation period ranges from two to fourteen days, averagely five days. It is possible to transmit the virus even if a person has no symptoms or before they develop symptoms (2 days before). The survival of the virus varies according to the surface: air 3hrs, copper 4hrs, cardboard 24hrs, stainless steel 72hrs, polypropylene 72hrs, on walls and floors 10 days.

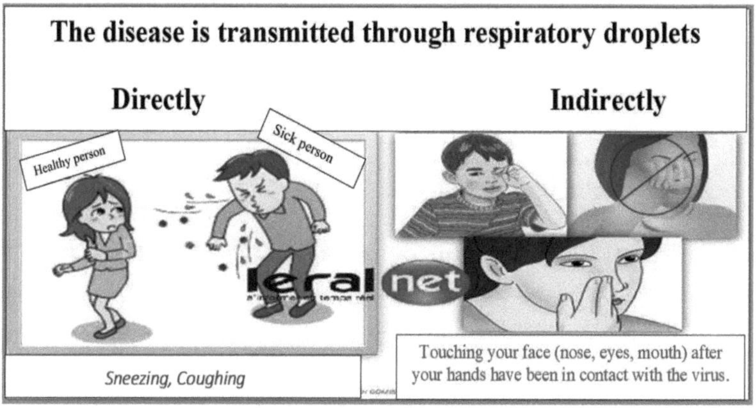

Figure: Coronavirus transmission

4. Clinical diagnosis

4.1. Risk factors

Everyone is at risk. Men are more affected than women. The following factors however, increase the risk of complications or severe forms:

1. Age extremes < 2 years, > 65 years;
2. Underlying diseases: diabetes, hypertension, cardiovascular disease, respiratory disease, kidney disease, liver disease, cancer, malnutrition, HIV, etc.;
3. Third trimester pregnancy;
4. Health and social workers.

4.2. COVID-19 signs and symptoms

Approximately 80% of infected persons are asymptomatic or have a mild form of influenza-like illness. Symptomatic patients without upper respiratory tract complications have: fever, asthenia, cough, malaise, body aches, sore throat, running nose, nasal congestion, headache, anosmia, agueusia, loss of appetite, diarrhoea.

Complications include breathing difficulties, intense fatigue, very high fever (39 °C), pneumonia, and kidney failure. Generally, 5-15% of patients develop severe forms of the disease. Its course cannot be predicted.

5. Para clinical diagnosis

The thoracic scan can be used to suggest a COVID-19 infection, but the definite diagnosis is carried out in the laboratory by nasopharyngeal sampling. Rapid diagnostic tests (RDT) are also available.

6. Prevention

- Regular hand washing with clean running water and soap or with alcohol-based solutions;
- Cough or sneeze into your elbow or into a disposable tissue;
- Use a disposable handkerchief and dispose of it in trash cans. If possible, use cleaning products to disinfect surfaces or objects (door handles, car steering wheel, motorbike handlebars, etc.) that may have been contaminated;
- Wear a suitable mask that covers the nose and mouth;
- Maintain a distance of at least 1.5m from anyone outside the house and from identified or suspected cases;
- Do not touch people when in public;
- Do not spit anyhow.

II. WATER, HYGIENE AND SANITATION

1. WASH norms and standards

1.1. Water requirement

Table: Norms and standards

Structures	Water requirement
Public toilets	1-2 litres per day per user for hand washing.
	2-8 litres per toilet block per day for cleaning.
Flush toilets	20-40 litres per user per day for flush toilets.
	3-5 litres per user per day for non-flush toilets.
Anal cleaning	1-2 litres per person per day.

1.2. Number of toilets needed for users

At least one toilet is needed for every 20-25 users. Urinals should also be provided in all men's toilet blocks, and bedpans for children under 7.

2. Application of standard precautions

2.1. Basic precautions

These are the precautions applicable to ALL at ALL times. They are the minimum preventive measures that apply at all times, to all people, regardless of their state. Risk assessment is essential for all activities; that is, assessing each activity and determining the personal protective equipment (PPE) needed for adequate protection.

2.2. Standard aspects of precautions

These include: hand hygiene, respiratory hygiene, risk-based PPE, prevention of accidents involving exposure to biological fluids, handling, cleaning and disinfection of common equipment and surfaces, environmental cleaning, safe handling and cleaning of soiled linen and waste management.

3. Hand hygiene

Hand hygiene is the best way to prevent the spread of germs in health care facilities and in the community. Our hands are our most important professional tool, playing a great role in the transmission chain. The guidelines of the World Health Organization (WHO) for hand hygiene are:

- Before cleaning an object or surface;
- After exposure to a biological fluid;
- Before and after any contact with objects or people,
- After contact with the surroundings of a sick person.

Hand hygiene requires the use of an appropriate product and technique. Alcohol-based sanitizer (preferably) can be used, if the hands are not visibly very dirty. Hands should be rubbed for 20-30 seconds or more if they are visibly dirty. Soap, running water and a disposable napkin may be used.

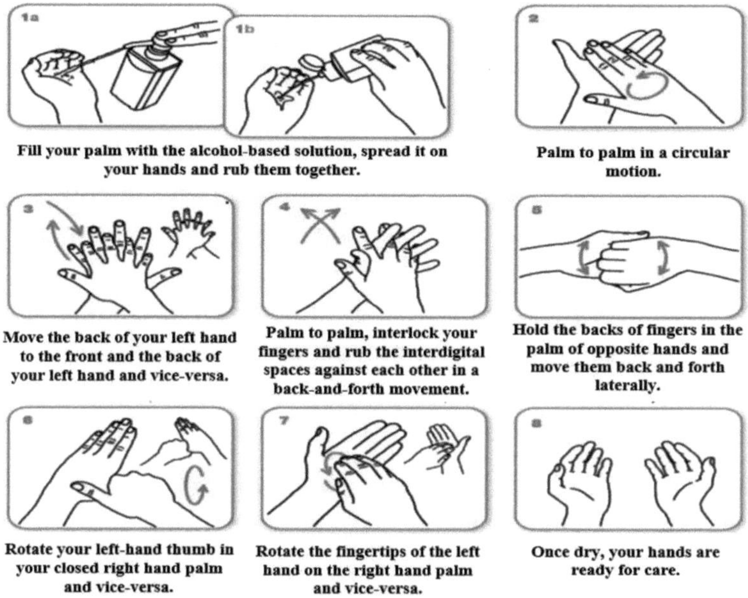

Figure: Hand hygiene with an alcohol-based solution

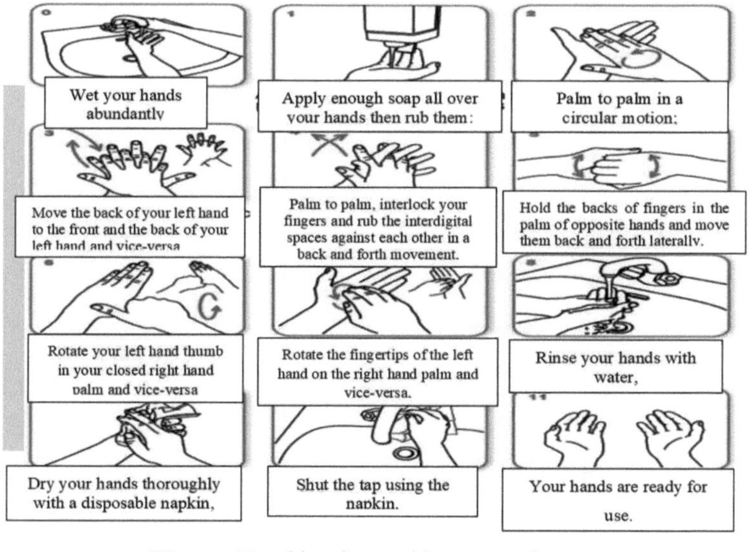

Figure: Hand hygiene with soap and water

4. Respiratory hygiene

Good respiratory hygiene can reduce the spread of micro-organisms that cause respiratory infections. Respiratory hygiene procedures include:

- Turning your head away from others when coughing or sneezing, or coughing into your elbow if a handkerchief is not available;
- Covering your nose and mouth with a handkerchief and disposing of it immediately in the trash can;
- Washing your hands with soap or an alcohol-based solution.

You also have to promote respiratory hygiene. That is, encourage hand washing for patients with respiratory symptoms, provide masks to all workshop/meeting participants, whether symptomatic or not. Also display visual aids reminding campers and visitors with or without respiratory symptoms to cover their coughs.

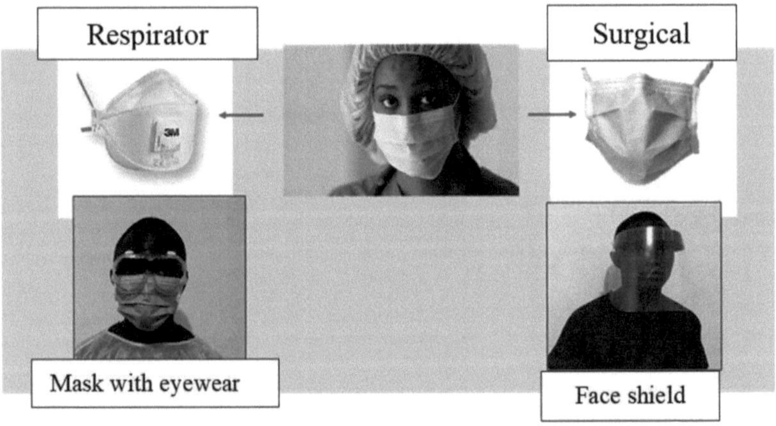

Figure: Types of face protection

3 **Wearing the mask** • Use a liquid-resistant, surgical or face shield mask • Cover your mouth, nose and chin • Adjust the flexible part of the nose • Keep it fit using the laces or buckles • Adjust it	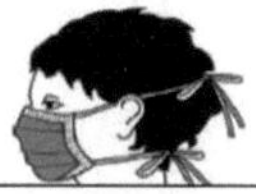 Procedure mask
Or a respirator • Choose the respirator that corresponds to your fit testing • Cover your nose, mouth and chin • Adjust the nosepiece on the nasal arch • Keep it tight using the upper and lower elastic strip • Adjust • Check the adjustment: 1. Inhale – The respirator should sag; 2. Exhale – Take note of any leaks around the face.	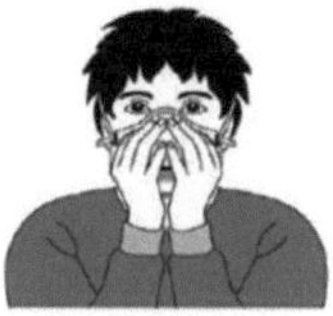 N95 or FFP2

***Figure*:** How to wear a mask or respirator

5. Personal Protective Equipment (PPE)

This is specialized attire or a device worn by health care workers to protect themselves when in contact with infectious agents. It provides protective barriers for the eyes, nose, mouth, skin, feet and clothing from contact with a patient's body fluids (blood, vomit, urine, faeces, sweat and pus). It is effective when used with other procedures and allows health care workers and visitors to carry out risky actions safely.

The principles of PPE use are: right size, secure, comfortable, stay in place without needing to be readjusted, caution when removing and handling PPE.

In order to know which PPE to don, a risk assessment must be carried out, and health care activities assessed to determine the appropriate personal protection. Risk assessment is the systematic examination of all labour aspects in order to evaluate the safety and health risks of staff and patients.

The effectiveness of PPE depends on regular and adequate supply, adequate staff training, good hand hygiene practices, appropriate behaviour in the isolation area (including use of PPE), and close supervision (in pairs) for donning and doffing PPE.

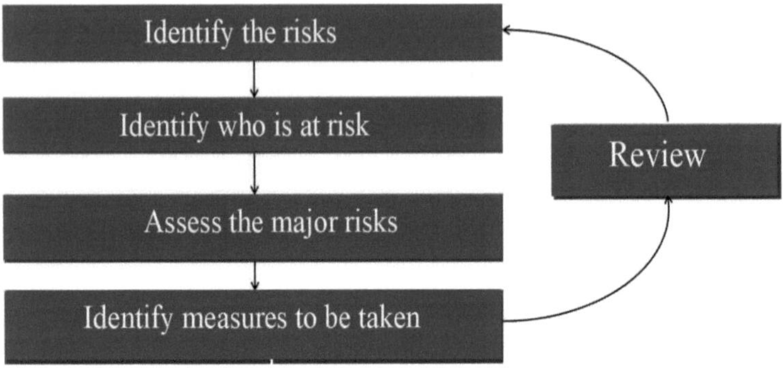

Figure: Risk assessment procedure

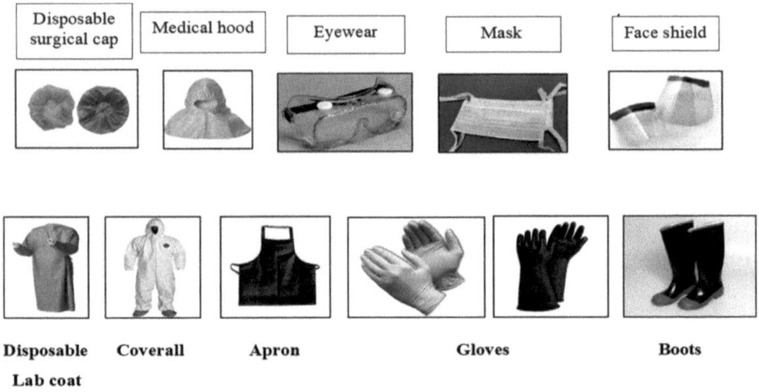

Figure: Personal Protective Equipment

5.1. Gloves

Health care gloves should be used in a number of clinical situations such as: exposure to blood, body fluids, secretions, excretions and equipment visibly soiled with body fluids; direct patient contact: contact with blood, mucous membrane, injured skin, suspicion of highly transmissible and pathogenic germs, epidemic or emergency situation, blood sampling, vascular opening, pelvic and vaginal examination, open system endotracheal aspirations.

Sterilized gloves are used for all surgical procedures, natural childbirth, invasive radiological procedures: insertion of vascular access (central line); preparation of complete parenteral nutrition and chemotherapeutic agents.

In addition, it is important to remember that wearing gloves does not replace hand hygiene, neither does it give allowance to have contact with PPE, or to pick up objects such as telephones, pens, books, patient files, etc. Gloves are not reusable.

Table: Glove wearing indications

	Information
Wearing of gloves	1) Before an aseptic procedure; 2) When contact with blood or another biological fluid is foreseen, including a case of contact with mucosa or abraded skin, irrespective of the need to create or maintain aseptic conditions; 3) In the event of contact with the patient (and his/her direct environment) when applying "contact" precautions.
Removal of gloves	1) Immediately the gloves are damaged or faulty (or that they seem not to be in good state); 2) Immediately it stops being in contact with blood, another biological fluid, abraded skin or mucosa; 3) Immediately it stops being in contact with a patient and his/her immediate environment or with a contaminated body; 4) When hand hygiene is required.

5.2. Boots and shoe covers

Boots or shoe covers should be worn when there is a risk of blood, body fluids or patient secretions splashing, spilling or dripping on your feet. Disposable shoe covers are mainly used in hospitals.

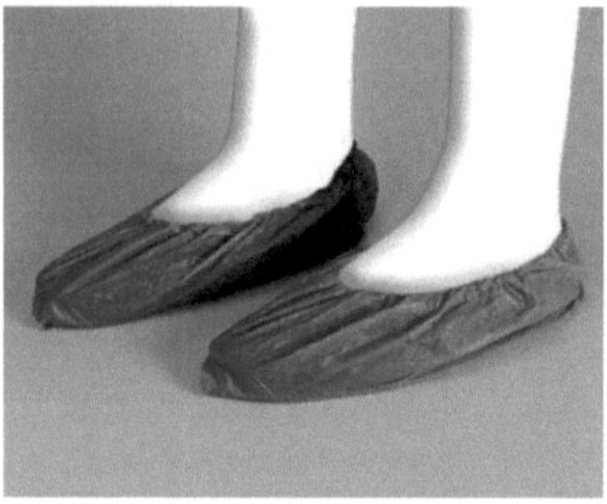

Figure: Disposable shoe covers

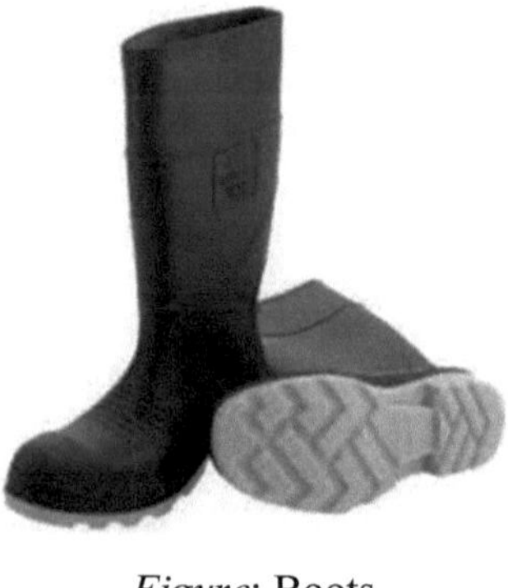

Figure: Boots

Always doff the PPE in the “PPE DOFFING ZONE” and obligatorily under the watch of a trained person. Whenever you doff a PPE, wash your gloved hands with 0.5% chlorinated water.

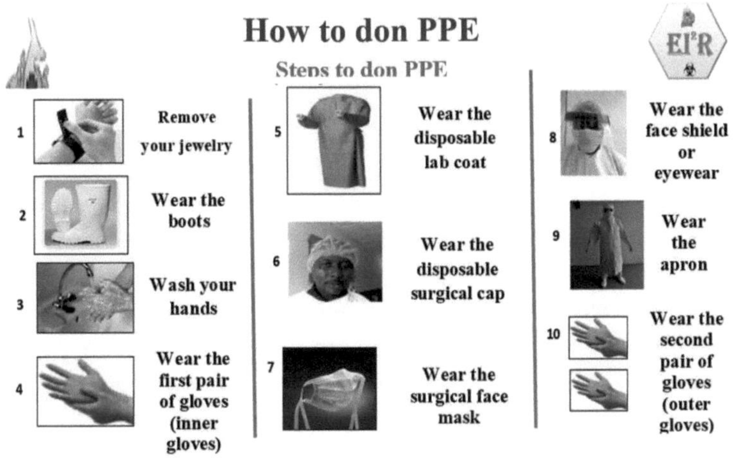

Figure: How to don PPE ?

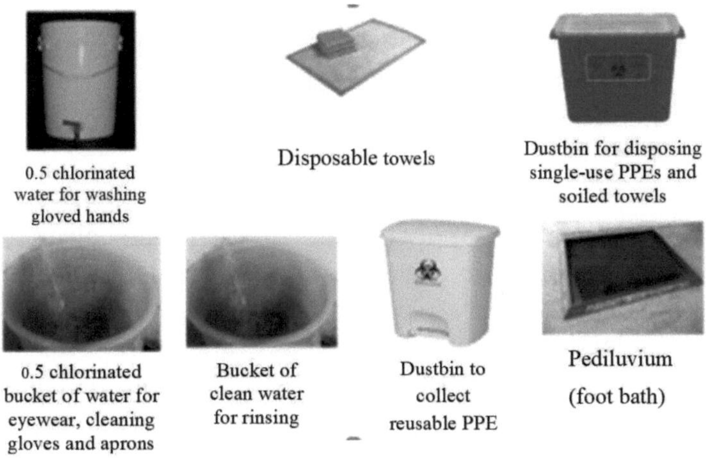

Figure: PPE material and doffing area

Table: Steps to doff extra PPE

1. Wash gloved hands (0.5% chlorinated water);	8. Wash your hands with the inner gloves (0.5% chlorinated water);	14. Wash your hands with the inner gloves (0.5% chlorinated water);
2. Remove outer gloves;	9. Remove outer surgical mask;	15. Remove inner gloves;
3. Wash your hands with inner gloves (0.5% chlorinated water);	10. Wash your hands with inner gloves (0.5% chlorinated water);	16. Wash your bare hands with water and soap or 0.5% chlorinated water;
4. Remove your apron;	11. Remove your disposable surgical cap;	17. Walk through a 0.5% chlorinated disinfection booth (pediluvium);
5. Wash your hands with inner gloves (0.5% chlorinated water);	12. Wash your hands with inner gloves (0.5% chlorinated water);	
6. Remove your eyewear or face shield;	13. Check your boots, disinfect them with a towel + 0.5% chlorine if necessary;	18. Remove your boots at the end of the day and wash your hands with water and soap or 0.5% chlorinated water.
7. Remove your lab coat. Wash your hands with the inner gloves (0.5% chlorinated water);		

6. Contact precautions to take in service

A note should be placed on each door and another on the file before coming in contact with the patient or his/her surroundings. Hand hygiene should be practiced, as well as wearing of gloves and a lab coat, and respect of the PPE doffing procedure (ThermoFlash, electronic tensiometer, glucometer, boots, visors and disposable lab coats) when possible.

The cleaner must apply isolation measures and clean the room at the end. Every visitor must wash their hands before and after the visit, wear procedure masks and ensure that they understand isolation measures and their reasons. Reception services must be notified before the patient is displaced.

7. How to isolate a patient?

1. ISOLATE the person with the symptoms;
2. INFORM the patient, his/her family and visitors. Make sure that they understand the isolation measures to take and their reasons;

3. PUT a note on the door or on the side of the bed;
4. LIMIT access to the family and visitors;
5. RESTRICT the patient's movements out of the room. If his/her displacement is necessary, inform the stretcher bearer and the receiving head of department.

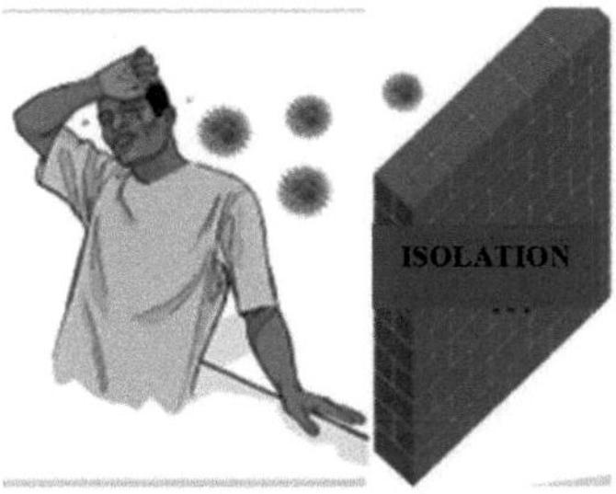

Figure: Isolation

8. How to take care of objects and surfaces?

8.1. Decontamination

This process consists in making an object or area safe by getting rid of dangerous micro-organisms or materials, and chemical, radioactive and infectious substances. Decontamination is important because it helps to reduce the spread of micro-organisms and other decontaminants which might affect the health of human beings. Micro-organisms can live on surfaces (tables, chairs), medical equipment (thermometer, stethoscope), in the air, in body fluids (droplets, blood, spittle, etc.)

8.2. Cleaning

This is the first necessary step to eliminate contamination by foreign bodies like dust or soil. It also helps to eliminate organic materials like blood, secretions, excretions and micro-organisms in order to prepare a surface for disinfection and sterilization.

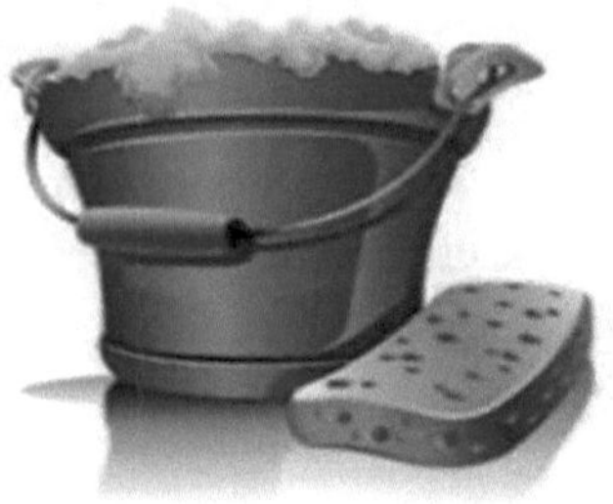

Figure: Mop bucket

8.3. Disinfection

This process is meant to reduce the number of active micro-organisms to a less harmful level. Nevertheless, it might not deactivate bacterial spores, prions and some viruses. Many products can be used as disinfectants, but chlorine is mostly used to disinfect surfaces. It is not recommended for instruments, medical equipment, electronic devices and non-water-resistant devices.

Here below are the principles for cleaning and disinfection:

- Always go from the cleanest to the dirtiest areas and from the highest to the lowest areas;
- Always clean and disinfect health care equipment for patients before use;
- Each task has a bucket for it; buckets meant for particular use must be labelled and/or given a specific colour;
- Isolation cleaning products must be preserved and used only for isolation.

NB: The isolation area must always be cleaned at the end.

Here are the steps for cleaning and disinfection:

- Carry out hand hygiene;
- Don PPE (gloves, waterproof lab coat, apron, boots, masks, protective eyewear or face shield) ;
- Take out garbage and dirty laundry;
- Clean and disinfect the area while following the 3-buckets technique. Always clean before disinfecting because using a disinfectant on a dirty surface kills the efficiency of the disinfectant;
- Let the surface dry out naturally;
- Empty the used buckets in the patient's toilet(s);
- Doff PPE following the technique;
- Carry out hand hygiene.

NB: Never spray disinfectant on the PPE and/or the clinical care areas whether they are taken or not.

Use a chlorine solution of 0.5% for disinfection. Be sure to respect the 10 minutes contact time between the surface and the chlorine solution (do not let it dry out). Never put a dirty towel in a bucket of chlorinated water because the water will be contaminated. Also, never wipe a surface with a dry towel (a dry towel spreads the debris or dirt instead of cleaning them).

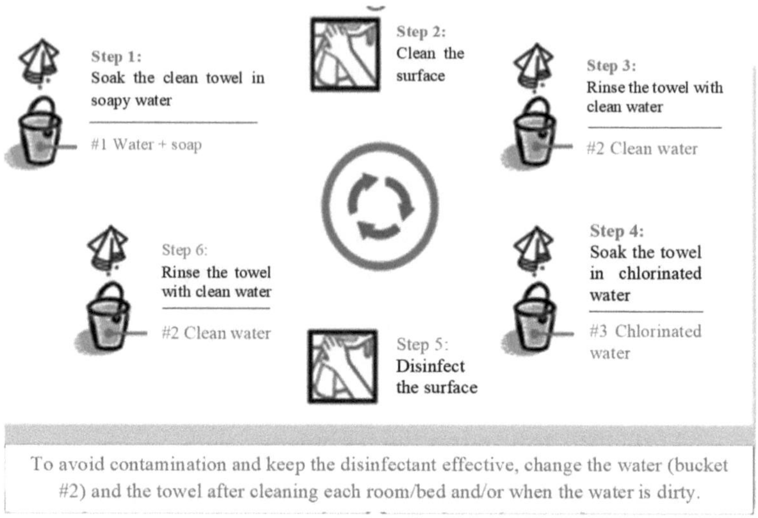

Figure: 3-buckets technique stage

8.4. Cleaning of body fluid spills

Follow the following steps: effect hand hygiene, don PPE, clean the spills with a cloth or a/an (paper) absorbent towel, immediately dispose of the cloth or towel in a plastic bag for infectious waste treatment, carefully clean it with a clean wet rag and neutral detergent (OMO, for example) or soap, rinse with clean water, disinfect, let the surface get dry and doff the PPE.

8.5. Disinfecting electronic instruments

They do not need to be cleaned before disinfecting. Wet the towel(s) and/or cloth(s) with 70% alcohol, wipe the instruments with this towel or cloth and let it/them get dry.

8.6. How to disinfect plates and utensils?

In order to disinfect plates and utensils: discard the leftover food, wash them with soapy water, rinse with clean water and allow to air-dry, wash the plates, cups and utensils with a (0.05%) chlorinated water solution and pour off the used chlorinated and soapy water in the patients' toilets.

8.7. How to clean reusable PPE ?

Collect the PPE (boots, cleaning gloves, aprons and eyewear), soak the PPE in a 0.2% chlorinated bucket of water for 10 minutes, remove the body fluids with clean water, wash with soapy water, then rinse with clean water, hang to dry, and lastly, pour off the chlorinated and soapy water in the toilet.

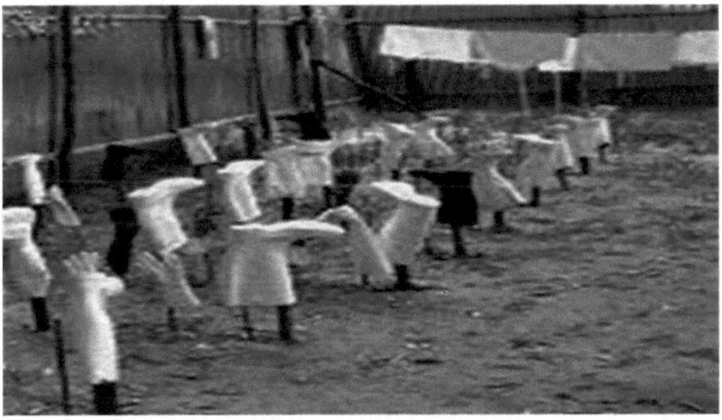

Figure: Drying of boots

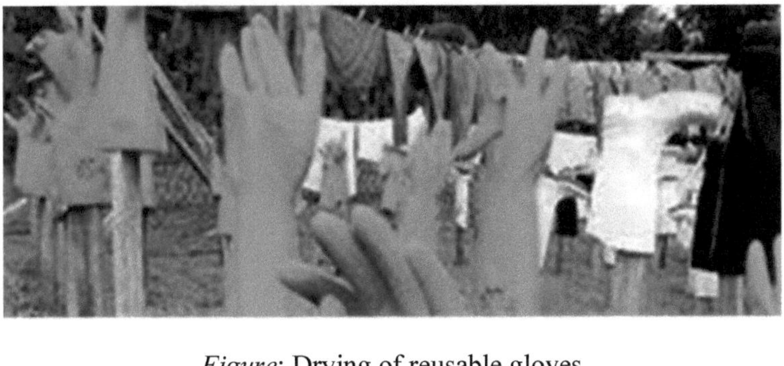

Figure: Drying of reusable gloves

8.8. How to wash the laundry ?

If there is solid dirt, fecal matter or vomit on the laundry, scrape it off with a solid and flat object, throw the waste in the patients' toilets and disinfect the container used. These are the steps to follow for washing laundry:

- Put the dirty linen in a container (a leak-free waterproof bag or bucket) before taking it out of the isolation area, and disinfect the outer part of the container;
- Take the container straight to the laundry room;
- Soak in 0.05% chlorinated water for **30 minutes**;
- Put the laundry in a tub of hot soapy water and shake it with a stick;
- Rinse with clean water;
- Spread for drying.

8.9. The footbath, or feet or shoe decontamination rag

Put a 2% chlorine solution, to be changed every 24 hours, at the entrance of camps, rooms or meeting rooms. Also put posters asking everyone to soak their shoes or legs inside before entry. If the water is too dirty before 24 hours, pour it off in the toilet and make more chlorinated water for the basin.

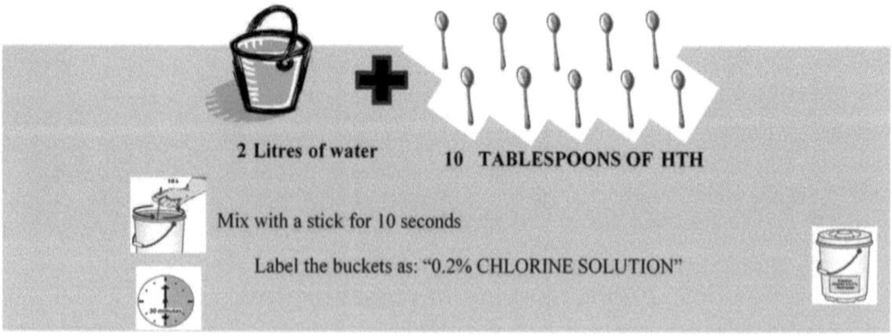

Figure: How to make a 0.2% chlorine solution with a 70% HTH?

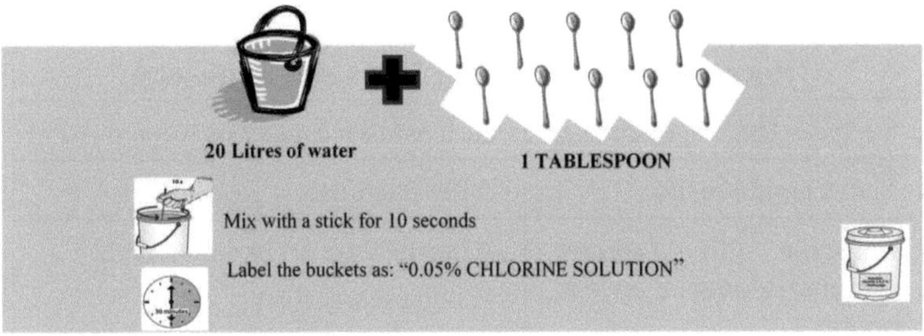

Figure: How to make a 0.05% chlorine solution with a 70% HTH?

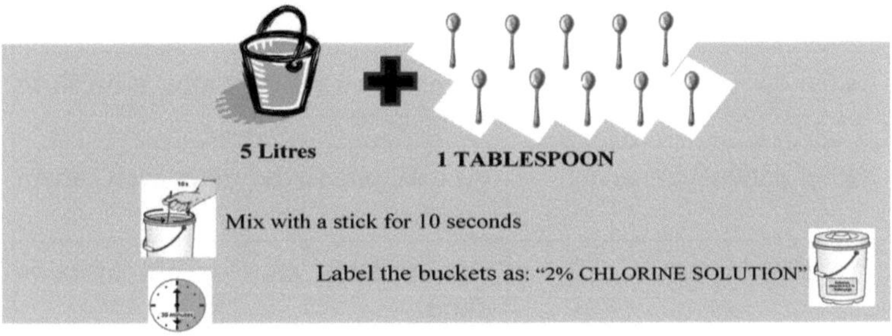

Figure: How to make a 2% chlorine solution with a 70% HTH?

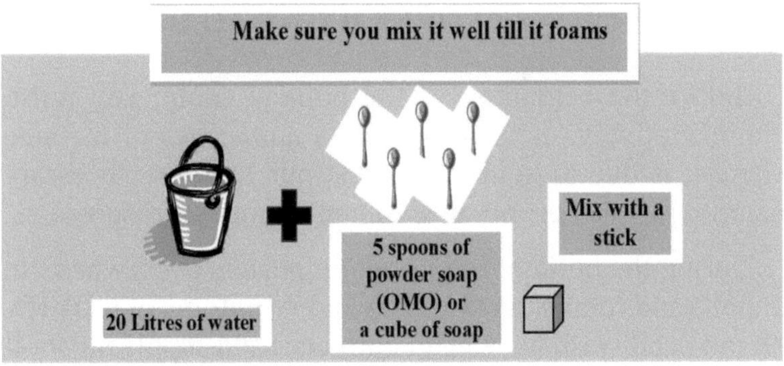

Figure: How to make soapy water

8.10. How to clean the waste buckets?

Wash them with soap and water, then rinse with warm water and, finally, rinse them with 0.2% chlorinated water.

Table: Cleaning frequency

Objects/areas	Cleaning frequency.
Surfaces (tables, chairs)	At least twice a day or when need be.
Plates and utensils	After each use.
Reusable PPE (aprons, cleaning gloves, eyewear, boots)	After leaving an isolation area; When clearly dirty; At the end of each day.
Medical equipment (ThermoFlash)	After each patient.
Isolation	At least once a day, after a break or when need be.
Other patient care areas	At least once a day, after each patient or when need be.
All the other areas	Immediately after a spill of body fluid

III. WHAT TO DO IN CASE OF COVID-19 SUSPICIONS. WHEN? WHAT TO DO?

Before the beginning of the holiday camp, you must, administratively, contact the health authorities of the area where it is due to hold. You must purchase the necessary material for the best practice of containment measures.

During the holiday camp: put up posters everywhere, in all halls and rooms, on the signs and symptoms of COVID-19; put hand wash tools at all entrances and supply alcohol-based solutions to halls or rooms, and necessary material for containment measures; take the temperature of each camper every day and at the beginning of each activity if need be; immediately call health authorities in case of illness, most especially if the patient is suspected of having COVID-19.

After the holiday camp, as a matter of obligation, give a report of the camp to the health authorities of the area.

Table: List of types of equipment and materials

TYPE	EQUIPMENT/MATERIALS
Personal protective equipment	Cleaning gloves Visors Surgical or filtration fabric masks Boots Disposable lab coats Health care gloves
Hand wash and cleaning tools	Buckets of different volumes (5l, 10l, 20l, 50l, 100l) Tap bucket Liquid soap Granular chlorine Alcohol-based solution (1 container per person per day) Powder soap
Waste management tools	Rag Footbath basin Buckets with lids Trash bags
Others	Backpack or manual sprayers Thermoflash Electronic tensiometer

CHAPTER IV

WHAT HAPPENS TO LEISURE AFTER THE COVID-19 PANDEMIC?

The COVID-19 pandemic has had, and may still have for a while, a negative impact at the socio-economic level and specifically on leisure. Rather than resign to it, it would be wise to focus on the lessons learnt from this health crisis. Actually, the lessons the COVID-19 pandemic has taught us, in terms of respect for hygiene and safety rules, must be capitalised even more widely in the organization of leisure activities. They should also spur us to devise new ideas for the development of the tourism and leisure sector.

How can we take advantage of the opportunities offered by the texts on decentralization to increase the provision of leisure activities? The process of decentralization ended with the election of regional councillors and the setting up of management teams. How will qualitative and quantitative leisure be offered to Cameroonians, with the devolution of powers to Regional and Local Authorities and the inclusion of the civil society? In an urge to accelerate decentralization and in view of the very high demand, the organization of leisure activities cannot remain the prerogative of the State and the lone ministry in charge of leisure activities. We should take advantage of the facilities which decentralization offers to revive the tourism and leisure sector.

I. ECENTRALIZATION: AN OPPORTUNITY

The new vision of leisure development is based on the coherence of the laws on decentralization and the texts governing tourism and leisure in Cameroon. It has been developed based on the shortcomings observed in the field and in response to the real needs of each local community according to the social utility criteria of available resources. Its primary objective is to widen the range of possibilities for accessible quality leisure activities adapted to the sometimes contradictory realities of different clienteles. Based on the pooling of efforts and a responsible distribution of roles, actions will be directed towards the increase of infrastructure, diversification of funding sources, training of stakeholders and the strengthening of the legal framework.

The new possibilities for the development of leisure activities are based on the coherence of the laws on decentralization and the texts governing tourism and leisure activities in Cameroon.

In accordance with Article 5 of Law No. 2016/006 of 18 April 2016 to regulate tourism and leisure activities in Cameroon: "The government, alongside the regional and local authorities, shall be responsible for implementing the national tourism and leisure policy."

Article 6 states that: "Every natural person or legal entity has the right to carry out tourism and leisure activities over the territory, pursuant to the laws and regulations in force, and the standards of professionalism recognized by international norms and standards."

Performance is the ultimate goal of any organization, and it is measured by relevance, effectiveness and efficiency. Relevance refers to the correctness, appropriateness and truthfulness of what it is all about.

Effectiveness refers to the production of expected results and effects. Lastly, efficiency consists in achieving the best results with the best means. One can conclude that the objective of any system of governance is performance. That is, the capacity to adequately meet public expectation. Specifically, what are the dividends to be drawn from the laws and other texts governing decentralization in the field of tourism and leisure?

That is the objective of this chapter, which will focus on the following points:

- The theoretical framework of decentralization;
- The situational analysis of leisure in Cameroon;
- The new leisure policy;
- The role of stakeholders in leisure policy.

In an urge to accelerate decentralization and in view of the very high demand, the organization of leisure activities cannot remain the prerogative of the State and the lone ministry in charge of leisure activities.

According to the terms of Article 2 (1) of Law No. 2004/17 of 22 July 2004 on the orientation of decentralization:

"Decentralization is the devolution of certain powers and appropriate means, by the State, to regional and local authorities. Decentralization is the main axis for promoting the development of democracy and good governance at the local level."

Article 10 of Law No. 2019/024 of 24 December 2019 to institute the general code of regional and local authorities stipulates that:

"Local authorities may, as part of their mandate, execute projects in partnership with one another, with the State, public establishments, semi-public, public and private enterprises, civil society organizations or foreign partners under the terms and conditions laid down by the laws and regulations in force."

Article 17 : "The State shall devolve, to local authorities, the powers necessary for their economic, social, health, educational, cultural and sports development."

Articles 5 and 6 of the 2016 Law on tourism and leisure activities state that "The government, alongside the Regional and Local Authorities, shall be responsible for implementing the national tourism and leisure policy... Every natural person or legal entity has the right to carry out tourism and leisure activities over the territory, pursuant to the laws and regulations in force, and the standards of professionalism recognized by the international norms and standards."

The new vision of leisure is conceived in response to the real needs of each local community according to the criteria of social utility of available resources. Its primary objective is to widen the range of possibilities for accessible quality leisure activities adapted to the sometimes contradictory realities of different clienteles.

It aims to:

- Contribute to economic development by promoting the emergence of a competitive private sector in tourism and leisure;
- Protect and preserve national cultural values through the promotion of healthy and educational leisure activities and to encourage the mixing of populations, national integration and togetherness;
- Encourage the building of adequate infrastructures and provision of services to enable young people to have access to sports, cultural, recreational and leisure activities;

- Build and provide leisure infrastructures and services in rural and urban areas;
- Train community leaders, starting with young people themselves, in the field of sports and leisure;
- Provide young people with equal access to sports and artistic activities and boost their creativity;
- Devolve powers to regions and municipalities and establish partnerships for leisure for all;
- Make leisure an essential component of policy responses to social demand in order to provide positive well-being and build a better future for mankind.

II. THE STRATEGIC AXES OF THE NEW VISION OF LEISURE

The revival of leisure activities involves capitalizing on the opportunities offered by decentralization and the lessons learnt from the COVID-19 pandemic. It is based on 5 major axes which are:

- Developing infrastructure;
- Strengthening regulation;
- Diversifying the financing of leisure activities;
- Developing human resources;
- Developing and promoting traditional leisure activities.

1. Developing infrastructure

The analysis of the situation revealed the lack of infrastructure for leisure activities, despite the relevant provisions of Articles 1 and 2 of the 1974 law which state that: “Any development project, school or university building project and realization of residential or industrial real estate project must include... land necessary for the installation of sports and socio-educational equipment... Any structure intended for sports and socio-educational leisure and outdoor activities shall be considered as sports and socio-educational equipment." It can be noticed that schools, residential areas and villages are seriously lacking leisure infrastructures.

In fact, few schools have any platforms for outdoor activities. In residential areas and villages, recreational activities take place on empty and disused land. Boarding schools capable of hosting holiday camps are becoming increasingly rare. Many tourist sites have no facilities to accommodate individuals and groups of people within the minimum terms and conditions of hygiene and safety.

In view of this situation, it is strongly recommended that efforts be directed towards the construction and rehabilitation of leisure facilities. These initiatives should be integrated into the construction of schools or residential quarters. It is just a matter of complying with the regulations in force.

Article 17 of Law No. 2019/024 of 24 December 2019 to institute the general code of regional and local authorities states that: "The State shall devolve to local authorities, the powers necessary for their economic, social, health, educational, cultural and sports development." Therefore, the construction of light and suitable infrastructure in each community can contribute to address the lack of leisure practice spaces.

Another alternative would be to pool the use of existing infrastructure according to a well-established programme and rules. For example, a classroom can be used for music lessons for idle youths after formal classes. Or a college field can be used by local football clubs over the weekend.

2. Strengthening regulations

It has been pointed out that the various initiatives taken in the context of leisure time organization do not respect the regulations in force. There is an old saying that: "ignorance of the law is no excuse". However, it is worth noting that there has been no implementing legislation on the 2016 law on tourism and leisure activities. In general, the law gives general guidelines. Specifications for public and private sponsors of activities of a sector are contained in the application texts. So, texts subsequent to the 2016 law really need to be available in order to clarify the responsibilities of the various tourism and leisure stakeholders. At national level, holiday camps are placed under the authority of the Ministry in charge of Tourism and Leisure. Its mission is to apply the changes desired by the legislator, draw up ad-hoc regulations, define the obligations of the organizers and set up tools for monitoring and evaluating the camps. The Ministry also has a role to promote holiday camps and ensure their development and educational quality.

3. Diversifying the financing of leisure activities

As of now, Government provides the bulk of funding for its leisure activities. Many ministries are involved in funding and organizing leisure activities. These include, but are not limited to, the Ministry of Tourism and Leisure, the Ministry of Arts and Culture, the ministries responsible for the various levels of education, etc.

Better coordination of leisure activities and pooling of resources could facilitate the organization of mass activities with a real impact on the target population. Regional and local authorities can undertake to finance certain projects. In any case, the law gives each community the free will to levy taxes on different activities deemed as priorities.

4. Developing human resources

The inadequacy of human resources in terms of quality and quantity has been identified as a limitation to the proper supervision of leisure activities. It is common to see gymnasiums or "health clubs" being transformed into torture centres due to the incompetence of supervisors. Some holiday camps lack pedagogical projects, simply because the supervisors think that the main thing is to make the children play.

For the past two years, the Ministry of Tourism and Leisure has been training leisure activity supervisors. About 200 people from MINTOUL, regional and local authorities and private sponsors have been trained. However, given the demand in the field, the number of supervisors has been ridiculous. To improve the ratio of supervisors to trainees, it would be very useful to increase the number of training sessions by deploying teams to the field.

5. Developing and promoting traditional leisure activities

Throughout Cameroon, and for many years now, there have been several traditional leisure activities within communities. Adults and children alike, men and women, individually or in groups, all practice these leisure activities. The activities help develop various faculties such as skill, attention, agility, memory development, endurance, expressions of female and male beauty, physical strength, etc. According to functions, one can distinguish between cerebral, gymnastic, artistic, epic, endurance, mystical, popular and initiatory games.

Among the best known of these various leisure activities can be cited for example, the *Tilé,* also called the *Songo* by other communities (token game), the *Mesiñ* (wrestling), the

Dingagana (tales, epics), the *assiko* (dance), the *Bolobo*, the *Njang* (Banso dance), the *Fantasia* (horse racing), the *Djâgue* (horse riding), the canoe race, the *Isoko* (beach game), swimming in the sea, river or marigot, the *Mendjan* (token game) etc.

The promotion of these traditional leisure activities has become, for the Ministry of Tourism and Leisure and all stakeholders of this sector, an emergency which involves many stakes not only for the national and global cultural heritage, but also and especially for the development and consolidation of the practice of leisure activities within the Cameroonian society, in the city as in the countryside, for the fulfilment of all walks of life.

Nonetheless, to achieve such a range of lofty goals, some prerequisites must be met, including the training of multisector human resources. It may be a daunting task, yet the Ministry of Tourism and Leisure has included the development and promotion of traditional leisure activities in its programme for the new vision of leisure.

III. SYNERGY OF COMPETENCES IN THE FIELD OF LEISURE

The new leisure policy, based on a judicious analysis of the texts in force, calls for a synergy of responsibilities between the Ministry of Tourism and Leisure, the Regional and Local Authorities and the Civil Society Organizations. Such a collaboration platform presupposes a proper distribution of roles to avoid possible conflicts and overlaps. Apart from specifying the role of each stakeholder, the action of the supervisory authority is expected to focus on the devolution of powers and advocacy for an increase in the supply of leisure activities.

1. The Ministry of Tourism and Leisure

Since the signing of Decree No. 2012/291 of 21 June 2012, the Ministry of Tourism and Leisure is recognised as the leading authority in leisure development. It is its responsibility to give the general guidelines, as well as the measures for monitoring and controlling activities in this sector. As such, it is responsible for:

- Defining sector policies and developing projects and programmes on leisure activities, including the training of various stakeholders;
- Developing draft texts and procedures and ensuring the control, monitoring and evaluation of programmes, projects and activities;
- Mobilizing human and financial resources and redistributing them;
- Initiating co-operation and collaboration strategies with the various partners;
- Identifying the powers to be devolved, as well as accompanying resources.

2. Regional and Local Authorities

Finalisation of the decentralization process shall give important responsibilities to councils and regions through the mechanism of devolution of powers. In this perspective, the regional and local authorities are called upon to:

- Popularize and apply and enforce the texts regulating leisure activities within their jurisdiction;
- Incorporate tourism and leisure programmes, projects and activities into local development plans;
- Create space for leisure activities and build local leisure facilities;

- Make an inventory of healthy leisure structures and activities;
- Promote traditional leisure activities and games;
- Create partnerships with private sponsors and councils given the context of decentralization;
- Identify the training needs of potential sponsors and organize training sessions for leisure activity and board game supervisors;
- Carry out awareness campaigns for the population on the therapeutic, social and economic values of leisure activities;
- Monitor the activities of local authorities and partners;
- Monitor and levy taxes on tourism and leisure activities.

It would not be superfluous to particularly stress the impact of leisure activities, especially holiday championships and youth work camps, on local development. In particular, voluntary youth work camps contribute greatly to the development of land use planning policies and allow the population to take part in them. The involvement of the local population, especially young people, is one of the desired goals in the implementation of labour-intensive work (HIMO). Championships and other festivals are also privileged moments for mobilizing young people around civic values and cultural heritage.

It is therefore necessary to provide information prior to the organization of the various activities. That is why it would appear advisable that leisure activities be included, as much as possible, in the local development initiative. In terms of strategy, the notions of consultation and pooling of synergies between the different stakeholders are essential.

3. Civil Society Organizations

Civil society organizations recognized by the Ministry of Tourism and Leisure are an important component in the development of leisure activities. To be able to play their role fully, they must:

- Acquire the regulations governing public policies on tourism and leisure;
- Participate and involve staff in training courses and seminars on staff capacity building;
- Build or develop leisure facilities, if possible, under the control of the regional and local authorities and the supervisory authority;
- Register leisure activities in accordance with the regulations;
- Organize leisure activities at the grassroots;
- Contribute to the development and implementation of leisure policies;
- Provide data to build the file of private leisure stakeholders (programmes and reports of activities).

CONCLUSION

Leisure has been gaining in importance since the Industrial Revolution and Cameroon has not been exempted from this trend. In fact, leisure has become part of civic rights in our country, contributing to economic and social development. The benefits of leisure activities on physical and mental health are increasingly recognized and their practice is becoming more democratic. In order to reap their full benefits, leisure activities must be organized in compliance with legislation in force, observing health and safety rules, and under the supervision of qualified staff.

Unfortunately, its organization and practice have suffered organizational and regulatory setbacks including non-compliance with rules and regulations, inadequate infrastructure and qualified staff and funding difficulties. The COVID-19 pandemic, with its range of containment measures, has aggravated the shortcomings observed in the development of this industry. The COVID-19 pandemic has had and might still have, for some time to come, a negative impact at the socio-economic level. Nevertheless, the pandemic may be praised for reminding the stakeholders of the tourism and leisure sector of the indispensable requirements regarding hygiene and safety in the organization of leisure activities.

Faced with this situation, the authors deemed it useful to humbly offer public and private sponsors of leisure activities practical recommendations, and possible solutions to get the sector out of the ambient pessimism linked to the COVID-19 crisis. The main recommendation is to explore the opportunities offered by the general code of decentralization for the revival of economic activities, particularly in the tourism and leisure sector. This revival shall require a sound and voluntary pooling of human, material and financial resources.

BIBLIOGRAPHY

Alain CORBIN, *L'Avènement des loisirs : 1850-1960, Paris,* Aubier, 1995

Joffre DUMAZEDIER, *Vers une civilisation du loisir ?* Paris, Le Seuil, 1962.

Laurent TURCOT, *Sports et Loisirs. Une histoire des origines à nos jours*, Paris, Gallimard 2016.

Paul YONNET, *Travail, loisir, Temps libre et lien social,* Paris, Gallimard, 1999.

- Law No. 74/22 of 5 December 1974 on sports and socio-educational facilities;
- Law No. 2004/17 of 22 July 2004 on the orientation of decentralization;
- Law No. 2016/006 of 18 April 2016 to regulate tourism and leisure activities in Cameroon;
- Law No. 2019/024 of 24 December 2019 to institute the general code of Regional and Local Authorities;
- Decree No. 2012/291 of 21 June 2012 to organize the Ministry of Tourism and Leisure;
- Order No. 2/CG/JS/EP of 15 February 1963 on the organization and operation of Holiday Camps in the Federal Republic of Cameroon.
- Standard precautions in health care: Aide-memoire, WHO Oct 2007. http://www.who.int/csr/resources/publications/EPR_AM2_E7.pdf

- Hand Hygiene: Why, How & When? http://www.who.int/gpsc/5may/Hand_Hygiene_Why_How_and_When_Brochure.pdf?ua=1
- My 5 Moments for Hand Hygiene. World Health Organization. http://www.who.int/gpsc/5may/background/5moments/en/
- Personal protective equipment for use in a filovirus disease outbreak Rapid advice guideline, OMS 2016. http://apps.who.int/iris/bitstream/10665/251426/1/9789241549721-eng.pdf?ua=1

TABLE OF CONTENTS

Structures éditoriales du groupe L'Harmattan

L'Harmattan Italie
Via degli Artisti, 15
10124 Torino
harmattan.italia@gmail.com

L'Harmattan Hongrie
Kossuth l. u. 14-16.
1053 Budapest
harmattan@harmattan.hu

L'Harmattan Sénégal
10 VDN en face Mermoz
BP 45034 Dakar-Fann
senharmattan@gmail.com

L'Harmattan Cameroun
TSINGA/FECAFOOT
BP 11486 Yaoundé
inkoukam@gmail.com

L'Harmattan Burkina Faso
Achille Somé – tengnule@hotmail.fr

L'Harmattan Guinée
Almamya, rue KA 028 OKB Agency
BP 3470 Conakry
harmattanguinee@yahoo.fr

L'Harmattan RDC
185, avenue Nyangwe
Commune de Lingwala – Kinshasa
matangilamusadila@yahoo.fr

L'Harmattan Congo
67, boulevard Denis-Sassou-N'Guesso
BP 2874 Brazzaville
harmattan.congo@yahoo.fr

L'Harmattan Mali
ACI 2000 - Immeuble Mgr Jean Marie Cisse
Bureau 10
BP 145 Bamako-Mali
mali@harmattan.fr

L'Harmattan Togo
Djidjole – Lomé
Maison Amela
face EPP BATOME
ddamela@aol.com

L'Harmattan Côte d'Ivoire
Résidence Karl – Cité des Arts
Abidjan-Cocody
03 BP 1588 Abidjan
espace_harmattan.ci@hotmail.fr

Nos librairies en France

Librairie internationale
16, rue des Écoles
75005 Paris
librairie.internationale@harmattan.fr
01 40 46 79 11
www.librairieharmattan.com

Librairie des savoirs
21, rue des Écoles
75005 Paris
librairie.sh@harmattan.fr
01 46 34 13 71
www.librairieharmattansh.com

Librairie Le Lucernaire
53, rue Notre-Dame-des-Champs
75006 Paris
librairie@lucernaire.fr
01 42 22 67 13